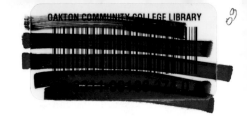

AIDS,
Drugs and Society

D1265313

AIDS, Drugs and Society

Edited by Anna Alexandrova

International Debate Education Association
NEW YORK ❖ AMSTERDAM ❖ BRUSSELS

Published in 2002 by
The International Debate Education Association
400 West 59th Street
New York, NY 10019

ISBN 0-9702130-2-6

Library of Congress Cataloging-in-Publication Data
AIDS, drugs, and society / edited by Anna Alexandrova.
    p.cm. -- (Sourcebook on contemporary controversies)
    Includes bibliographical references.
    ISBN 0-9702130-2-6
    1. AIDS (Disease) -- Prevention. 2. Intravenous drug abuse -- Health
aspects. 3. Narcotic addicts--Health and hygiene. 4. Narcotics addicts--
Diseases. I. Alexandrova, Anna, 1976- II. Series.

RA643.8 .A43 2002
614,5'99392--dc21   2002022156

Printed in the United States of America

The International Debate Education Association (IDEA) has dedicated itself to building open and democratic societies through teaching students how to debate. The IDEA Sourcebooks on Contemporary Controversies series is a natural outgrowth of that mission. By providing students with books that show opposing sides of hot button issues of the day as well as detailed background and source materials, the IDEA Sourcebooks on Contemporary Controversies give students the opportunity to research issues that concern our society and encourage them to debate these issues with others.

IDEA is an independent membership organization of national debate programs and associations and other organizations and individuals that support debate. IDEA provides assistance to national debate associations and organizes an annual international summer camp. Since 1994 IDEA has introduced debate to secondary schools and universities throughout Central and Eastern Europe, the former Soviet Union, Central Asia and Haiti and continues to grow throughout the world.

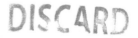

Table of Contents

Introductory Essay

I t has been twenty years since the Morbidity and Mortality Weekly published a Centers for Disease Control report on a mysterious outbreak of *Pneumocystis Pneumonia* in Los Angeles.[1] The report suggested the possibility of a cellular-immune dysfunction[2] related to a common exposure that would predispose individuals to opportunistic infections such as *pneumocystis carnii pneumonia*.[3] It was a symptom of a new disease, now known as AIDS, acquired immune deficiency syndrome. Since the epidemic began, over 18 million lives have been claimed by AIDS – almost 15 million of them in sub-Saharan Africa.[4] The AIDS toll can be expected to double over the next decade since over 34 million people are now estimated to be living with HIV or AIDS, and around five million new infections occur annually.[5] The disease has stricken different countries around the world, as well as different communities. In the United States some 800,000 to 900,000 people of all ages, ethnicities and sexual orientations are living with the virus.[6] Since June 5, 1981, AIDS has killed more than 438,000 people. In the US, the disease control agency estimates, as many as 900,000 people are infected with HIV[7]. Of these, 320,000 have developed AIDS, which occurs when the virus debilitates the immune system enough to make patients vulnerable to a range of other infections. Each year, federal health officials say, another 40,000 Americans become infected with HIV.[8] By the end of the year 2000, 36,1 million people worldwide were living with HIV/AIDS, 90 per cent in developing countries and 75 per cent in sub-Saharan Africa.[9]

These numbers are indeed alarming, however, they are likely to fall short of revealing the true severity of the problem. Many countries are faced with another epidemic that fuels the fast spread of

HIV/AIDS: drug use. It is well known that HIV is a blood-borne infection and can be easily transmitted from an infected user through drug injection equipment to the next user of the equipment. This can happen under several circumstances: sharing of a needle or other injection paraphernalia, re-use of a syringe, or non-sterile drug preparation.[10] In other words, the infection among this group of population spreads through specific actions that can be detected and prevented.

This manual introduces a reader to one pragmatic public health approach to disease prevention - harm reduction. There is no agreement on the correct definition of the term, its nature seems to be quite broad, but many agree that it means a policy aimed at reducing adverse consequences of drug use, "while the user continues to use drugs".[11] The approach itself is nothing new, but rather an extension of already existing ones, with a focus on pragmatism and cost-effectiveness.[12] Programs aimed at reduction of drug-related harm and prevention of further transmission of HIV and other blood-borne diseases have been subjects for a widespread discussion over the last 15 years. They were implemented and terminated,[13] praised and condemned,[14] and evaluated with different outcomes.[15] Despite the consensus of many professionals in different fields (such as: medical, public health, social, legal, etc) about the importance of the intervention and its effectiveness in reducing exposure to unnecessary risk, in the United States[16] needle exchange programs are not federally funded, and several attempts were made to pass relevant legislation forbidding this funding in the future.[17]

Harm reduction programs, which included needle and syringe exchange (NEP), outreach work and referral to medical institutions, originating in Europe, were successfully introduced to many countries in the world (US, Canada, Brazil, Europe, countries of Eastern Europe and Central Asia), when the methadone maintenance therapy[18] is politically acceptable only in some of them. Despite direct recommendations for the interventions from these international health agencies,[19] the projects still have to overcome difficulties in their everyday operations due to the barriers created by existing drug policies and, in some instances, indifference on the governmental level.

In order to start debating around the importance of harm reduction interventions, the first issue that one has to determine is whether it is necessary at all to pay any attention to drug injectors and to define their role in the spread of the epidemic. If such attention is important, then the question naturally arises: what would be the best way to prevent the spread of HIV through drug use? In order to help the reader answer this and other questions, the first part of the volume consists of essays on the background information and historical aspects of the HIV/AIDS epidemic.

The introductory section begins with an essay by Pat O'Hare and Diane Riley where the authors lay out different approaches to the issue of harm reduction, its main characteristics and its brightest examples. It is followed by an extract from Lawrence Gostin's work *The Interconnected Epidemics of Drug Dependency and AIDS*, where he explains why needle sharing fuels HIV/AIDS epidemics, and why it is a public health problem of such broad dimensions. Despite the fact that the essay was written ten years ago and described the situation in the US at the time, the article is extremely useful even nowadays as it provides the reader with solid legal and public health reasoning about HIV/AIDS epidemic among intravenous drug users (IDUs). With the fast growth of drug use and needle-borne spread of HIV the author concludes that the "war on drugs" was not successful, despite tremendous governmental efforts to curb the drug dependency. He offers different strategies for controlling the spread of HIV in the drug-dependent population that are consistent with the idea of reducing drug-related harm.

The consensus statement from the US National Institutes on Health follows the L. Gostin extract. In 1997 the US Institutes on Health came together for a panel discussion to weigh the scientific evidence and develop a draft consensus statement that included the following issues: identifying risky behavior and communities at risk for HIV; debating whether a reduction in these behavioral risks would lead to a decrease in the spread of HIV; and deciding what

would be the most effective way to implement risk-reduction procedures.[20] This consensus statement dissolves the fears that needle
exchange promotes drug use and increases the number of discarded
needles in the community. At the same time, the statement under-
lines the importance of drug abuse treatment as a central bulwark
in America's fight against AIDS. The section is completed by a
short extract from *HIV/AIDS and the Drug Culture: Shattered Lives*
that provides the reader with an excellent description of the four
most widely used models to control illicit behavior, such as drug
use.

Parts Two and Three of the book provide the substantive issues
for the debate. Part Two is dedicated to different policy aspects. It
begins with a general description of the past and current policies to
address illicit drug use. Michael Gossop presents the reader with
the digression into philosophy of freedom and the collision
between state's interest and the interest of an individual. He
describes the prohibitionist's control policies that were used
towards alcohol and other drugs at different times in the history of
Great Britain and the United States, and suggests some reasonable
alternatives to the policies of total prohibition and punishment of
the users. Robert DuPont and Eric Voth have a completely different point of view on the issue. The authors believe in the necessity of drug wars and cost-efficiency of a restrictive drug policy. They
advocate for a "strong" national policy that should reduce harm
through harm prevention, by creating drug abuse prevention programs and harm elimination, by implementing broader interdiction
and rehabilitation efforts.[21] Alex Wodak in his work opposes this
theory arguing its ineffectiveness due to the enormity of health
costs associated with illicit drug use and the inefficiency of supply
reduction policies as the only health choice available to drug users.
He argues that prohibition can be a successful policy where demand
is modest, domestic productions are difficult and other pshycho-
active substances are more readily available.

While policy is the main focus of Part Two, Part Three looks
into rights and legal aspects of the issue, specifically the interaction

of drug use, HIV and human rights. The human rights aspect of HIV/AIDS prevention seems to have gained its recognition within the last decade, and the importance of this interconnection was once again underlined during the UN Special Session on HIV/AIDS:

> The extent to which human rights are neglected or promoted is a major factor in the distribution of human immunodeficiency virus (HIV) within the population and the speed with which infection progresses to acquired immune deficiency syndrome (AIDS) and death.[22]

The first essay looks at drug use through a human rights perspective. Unfortunately, little is written about drug use and human rights, and the only international document that directly addresses drug users is the UN Convention Against Illicit Traffic in Narcotic Drugs and Psychotropic Substances. The only mention of human rights in this Convention can be found in Article 14, para 2, which speaks about measures designed to eradicate illicit cultivation of and demand for narcotic drugs and psychotropic substances, where the Convention mentions state's responsibility to respect fundamental human rights. The author of the piece presented for discussion (Norbert Gilmore) looks at the impact of the drug control measures on human rights, and more specifically, on the different aspects of the right to privacy, as the privacy implications of drug control measures are often overlooked. This leads to vulnerability from human rights abuses, as well as diminished capacity to exercise rights due to a number of social factors (the self-perception, stigma, criminalization of drug using behavior). The author concludes that improving the health of drug users by respecting their rights is possible, but such a policy would require a long-term commitment from the government and a shift in the policy that will include considering drug use as a risky, but not necessarily harmful, private activity.

In the following think piece, Ronald Bayer opens a discussion around HIV/AIDS exceptionalism. Bayer was one of the first to challenge the doctrine of HIV/AIDS exceptionalism in the early

1990s, when he had strongly opposed the theory that AIDS was different, and thus should be treated differently from both, social and legal perspectives.[23] He had argued that since the panic of mid-80s had passed, AIDS lost its salience as a public issue. In the presented article Bayer reaffirms his point of view through detailed analyzes of public health policy with regards to HIV testing of newborns and pregnant women, name reporting and access to public health care. He concludes that even if one does accept the uniqueness of HIV/AIDS as a disease, the necessity of the exceptional policy is highly debatable, as "the uniqueness of AIDS benefits renders them politically vulnerable",[24] especially in a profoundly unequal health care system.

Michael Closen in *The AIDS Epidemic as a Human Rights Challenge* represents a drastically different point of view from the one supported by Ronald Bayer. Closen argues that HIV/AIDS is an exceptional disease, thus it should be treated exceptionally. Indeed, HIV is a unique virus. It is lethal and is transmitted in ways that were usually scrutinized by the public. It affects people in their reproductive and most productive years. The disease mostly hits those who are already poor and socially unprotected, or isolated and discriminated against. Recently, scientists as well as AIDS activists, started thinking that twenty years after the virus was discovered and ten years after the new drugs became available, HIV and AIDS should not be treated exceptionally any longer. Thus, the state should be able to use its power in order to control the virus in the manner other diseases are being dealt with.[25] Some argue that there should not be any specific legislation protecting individuals with HIV, as there is none for those with cancer and heart disease. The presented essay explains the danger of this policy and comes to the conclusion that undressing HIV of its exceptional medical, social, ethical and legal status could be equal to the denial of the problem, and would result in disregarding its dramatic consequences.

In the next article, Scott Burris presents another approach to the theory of exceptionalism as beneficial to neither the people, affected by it, nor to public health policy. He argues that it is just an "-ism", an enemy ideology that discriminates against people living with AIDS (PLWAIDS). He suggests a rule of non-discrimination that will normalize a more quantitative approach to assessing risk in one's behavior. He concludes by noting the importance of de-emphasizing the difference between communicable and non-communicable health threats.

Part Four of the volume consists of the sources that the reader might find helpful in order to build up a fully informed discussion on the issue. It consists of some examples from the existing harm reduction programs, as well as Human Rights Treaties and documents that might be relevant for the debate.

The section opens with a review of the existing HIV prevention interventions among IDUs that are currently available and implemented in different countries of the world as well as have proven to be effective. The authors (Abu Abdul-Quader, Don Des Jarlais, Anindya Chatterjee, Elizabeth Hirky, Samuel Friedman) come up with a brief summary of some of these interventions and back up their findings with the experiences from Asia and Latin America. The purpose of this essay is to give the reader a perception of existing interventions and show that they worked not only in the countries of Western Europe and North America, but in countries with far more limited resources for its prevention. These interventions include: education of IDUs, increasing availability of clean injection equipment, decontamination of used needles and syringes, pharmacological treatment of drug addiction, outreach work. The extract addresses some issues in HIV prevention, looks into the effectiveness of each of the methods and opens a discussion on their importance and timely implementation.

The authors of the next article (Gemma Cox, Marie Lawless, Sean Cassin, Tighe Geoghegan) demonstrate the public health effectiveness of syringe exchange as a pragmatic response to drug use. They present the results of the first Irish follow-up study to establish the effectiveness of the above-mentioned intervention. The research outlines the following areas of the project's effectiveness: delivering basic services, improving access to sterile injection equipment, reducing the levels of infection and changing the risky injection behavior. They come to the conclusion that the syringe exchange programs can be highly effective as a public health initiative, as the availability of sterile injection equipment impacts the levels of sharing. However, there is still place for improvement, as the results of the study suggest lesser changes in risky sexual behavior. The Human Rights part of the Sources consists of extracts from basic human rights treaties, which are relevant to HIV/AIDS and the harm reduction approach. It opens with the most recent document - the UN Declaration of Commitment on HIV/AIDS "Global Crisis – Global Action", that was adopted during the Special Session on HIV/AIDS that took place June 25 – 27, 2001. It recognized the importance of HIV prevention, noting that it should be the mainstay of the national, regional and international response to the epidemic. It underlined that HIV prevention would include behavioral change as well as access to treatment, injecting equipment, condoms, lubricants, etc. Other documents and treaties presented in the manual in part provided a general framework for understanding of states' obligations with regards to HIV/AIDS and led to the adoption of the Declaration of Commitment.

A number of international human rights instruments relate to the disease in a general manner. These include: The Universal Declaration of Human Rights (1948), The International Covenant on Civil and Political Rights (1976), The International Covenant on Economic, Social and Cultural Rights (1976), The European Convention for the Protection of Human Rights and Fundamental Freedoms, Convention on the Elimination of All Forms of Discrimination Against Women (1979).[26] The International Guidelines on HIV/AIDS Prevention (included in the Sources part of the manual) were among the first documents to recognize the importance of HIV prevention through observance of human rights. These Guidelines are a consultation paper that was drawn up by a group of thirty-five experts in the field of HIV and human

rights, who outlined the various international human rights obligations that related to HIV. They emphasize the importance of
avoiding coercive and punitive measures with respect to HIV prevention, and suggest the prevention programs be designed in a
manner consistent with universally recognized human rights standards. Guideline 3 specifically addresses the above-discussed
exceptional character of HIV/AIDS by saying that it needs different provisions from those applicable to casually transmitted diseases. Guideline 4 reminds the law-makers about the need to
ensure that criminal legislation relating to the disease is consistent
with the international obligations of the country and are not misused or targeted against vulnerable groups. The comment to this
guideline addresses criminal law and its possible effects on the operation of needle exchange projects, and defines the issues that the
local legislation needs to address in order for harm reduction projects to operate effectively.

Unlike other international documents, presented in this part,
the Guidelines do not enjoy the legal status of a treaty and are not
binding to the State Parties. Their goal is to assure better understanding and implementation of human rights obligations.
However, the International Guidelines represent an important
document that is likely to be used once an HIV/AIDS related com-
plaint is brought for the consideration of the Human Rights
Committee or any other legal mechanism. They also provided the
developers of the UN Declaration of Commitment with some
background material on the State Parties' obligations.

As the presented articles will demonstrate, despite the long existence of harm reduction strategies and their acceptance within the
international community, the discussions around their importance,
applicability and legality have never stopped. The existing international instruments were used to help advocate for the strategies as
well as to abolish them. Still there are a lot of questions that have
to be answered: for example, despite one's right to the highest
attainable standard of health, in many countries drug users have no
access to methadone maintenance therapy, or any other substitu-

tion therapy, and some countries still hesitate to officially declare needle exchange as their public health policy. Harm reduction raises some difficult questions, but "it is obvious that debating these questions openly is better than ignoring them as has been done all too often in the past".[27] It is the hope of the editor that this manual will assist you in this important debate.

Anna Alexandrova
February 2002

NOTES

[1] *"Pneumocistys Pneumonia – Los Angeles"*, MMWR, June 5, 1981, 30:250-2.
[2] Immune response that involves enhanced activity by phagocytic cells and does not imply lymphocyte involvement. The definition is taken from *Online Medical Dictionary*, . Last revisited August 2, 2001 (herinafter referred to as the Online Medical Dictionary).
[3] Pneumocystis carinii is a microogranism that grows rapidly in the lungs of patients with immunosuppression, particularly due AIDS and is a leading AIDS-related case of death. *Online Medical Dictionary*, ibid.
[4] *AIDS and Population*, UNAIDS, http://www.unaids.org/fact_sheets/files/
[5] Ibid
[6] Villarosa, L, *One Diseases: Six Different Ways*, New York Times, June 5, 2001, available at: http://www.nytimes.com/pages/health
[7] Up to date surveillance data is available at: http://www.cdc.gov/hiv
[8] Ibid.
[9] UN Declaration of Commitment on HIV/AIDS, Global Crisis – Global Action, June 27, 2001. http://www.unaids.org/whatsnew/..._special/. Law visited July 24, 2001.
[10] Bourgois, P, *The Moral Economies of Homeless Heroin Addicts: Confronting Ethnography, HIV Risk, and Everyday Violence in San Francisco Shooting Encampments*, 33 SUBSTANCE ABUSE& MISUSE, (1998), 2323.
[11] See, for example, Bunning, E, Presentation made at St.Lawrence Forum on harm reduction, (March 1993), Toronto, 1. O'Hare, P, Riley, D. *Harm Reduction: History, Definition, and Practice*, in Harm Reduction: National and International Perspectives, Sage Publications, INC, Thousands Oaks, 2000, 8.
[12] Conley, P, et al, *Harm Reduction: Concepts and Practice*, (1998), available online:
[13] Broadhead, R, *Termination of an Established Needle-Exchange: A Study of Claims and Their Impact*, 46 SOC. PROBS, (1999), 48, 61.
[14] Voth, E, Levitsky, M, *Contemporary Drug Policy: Drug Policy Options*, NORTH-WEST. UNIV. J. INTERN'L POL'Y, 21/01/2000.
[15] Holtgrave, D, et al, *Cost and Cost-Effectiveness of Increasing Access to Sterile Syringes and Needles as an HIV Prevention Internvention in the United States*, 18 ACQUIR.IM. DEF. SYN. & HUM.RETROVIR., (Supp. I, 1998), S 133;

Bruneau, J, et al, *High Rates of HIV Infection Among Injection Drug Users Participating in Needle Exchange Programs in Montreal: Results of a Cohort Study*, 146 AM. J. EPID., (1997), 1007-1010.

[16] *National Institutes of Health Consensus Development Conference Statement, February 11 – 13, 1997*, as published in AIDS 2000, 14 (Supp. II), S 85 – 95.

[17] Geyser, D, *Needle Exchange Program Funding*, 37 HARVARD J. on LEGISLATION, winter 2000, 265.

[18] Maintenance treatment attempts to replace more dangerous illegal drugs with safer ones that are medically prescribed. "Maintenance can interrupt the progressively worsening processes of addiction by permitting the drug-dependent individual to end his or her reliance on illicit drug markets (with all their dangers), and it can effectively neutralize the most negative physiological aspects of addiction – the endless cycles of craving and avoidance of withdrawal." (Drucker, E, From Morphine to Methadone: Maintenance Drugs in the Treatment of Opiate Addiction, in Harm Reduction: National and International Perspectives, supra note 12, 33. Methadone is a synthetic drug that has similar molecular structure to heroin, and thus it is prohibited for use and circulation in many countries.

[19] Dr. Gro Harlem Brundtland, Director-General World Health Organization, Moscow, 2 November 2000, *Address to the Russian Academy of Medical Science*, ; *UNAIDS Task Force on HIV Prevention Among Injection Drug Users in Eastern Europe Progress Report*, supra note 12.

[20] Interventions to Prevent HIV Risk Behaviors, National Institutes of Health Consensus Development Conference Statement, February 11 – 13, 1997, published in AIDS 2000, Vol. 14 (Supp.2), S85-95.

[21] DuPont, R & Voth, E, Drug Legalization, Harm Reduction, and Drug Policy, Annals of Internal Medicine, (1995),123 (6): 461-465.

[22] UN Special Session on HIV/AIDS, Roundtable on HIV/AIDS and Human Rights.

[23] See Bayer, R, *Public Health Policy and the AIDS Epidemic: An End to HIV Exceptionalism?* New England J. Med.,(1991), 324: 1500.

[24] Bayer, R, *Clinical Progress and the Future of HIV Exceptionalism*, Archives of Internal Medicine, (24 May, 1999), 159 (10): 1042-48.

[25] See, for example, H.Fernandez, *Is AIDS Different?* Albany Law Review, 61 (3): 1073.

[26] Majority of the countries of the Eastern Europe and the Central Asia are parties to more than one of these international treaties. The full list of signatories to different conventions is available at: http://un.org

[27] See O'Hare & Riley, Harm Reduction: History, Definition, and Practice.

Part 1
Background readings concerning intravenous drug use and HIV

Harm Reduction: History, Definition and Practice

by Diane Riley Assistant Professor of Medicine,
University of Toronto & Pat O'Hare Executive Director
International Harm Reduction Association

*What do we mean when we say "harm reduction"?
Sometimes the approach is referred to as "harm
minimization" or "risk reduction". It represents both a goal
(the reduction of the number of harms associated with drug
use) and a strategy (a specific public health approach that
focuses on the negative consequences of drug use, rather than
on the use of illicit substances itself). It consists of five
components: pragmatism, focus on the human rights of drug
users, focus on harms, the need to balance costs and benefits
and hierarchy of goals. The roots of harm reduction are in
Europe, where it is recognized as an effective model in
countries like United Kingdom, the Netherlands,
Switzerland. Its practice includes a variety of measures
from needle exchange to peer support and drug
substitution therapy.*

First, do no harm.

-Hippocrates

THE NATURE AND ORIGINS OF HARM REDUCTION

Harm reduction is a relatively new social policy with respect to drugs that has gained popularity in recent years-especially in Australia, Britain, and the Netherlands as a response to the spread of Acquired Immune Deficiency Syndrome (AIDS) among injection drug users. This chapter provides an overview of the origins, background, and nature of harm reduction and some detailed examples of harm reduction as it is being practiced around the world.

Although harm reduction can be used as a framework for all drugs, including alcohol, it has primarily been applied to injection drug use (IDU) because of the pressing nature of the harm associated with this activity. The main focus of this chapter is the reduction of injection drug-related harm, although brief mention is made of alcohol and other noninjection drugs. Barriers to the adoption of harm reduction, as well as its limitations, are also discussed.

Harm reduction has as its first priority a decrease in the negative consequences of drug use. This approach can be contrasted with abstentionism, the dominant policy in North America, which emphasizes a decrease in the prevalence of drug use. According to a harm reduction approach, a strategy that is aimed exclusively at decreasing the prevalence of drug use may only increase various drug-related harms, and so the two approaches have different emphases. Harm reduction tries to reduce problems associated with drug use and recognizes that abstinence may be neither a realistic nor a desirable goal for some, especially in the short term. This is not to say that harm reduction and abstinence are mutually exclusive but only that abstinence is not the only acceptable or important goal. Harm reduction involves setting up a hierarchy of goals, with the more immediate and realistic ones to be achieved in steps on the way to risk-free use or, if appropriate, abstinence; consequently, it is an approach that is characterized by pragmatism.

Harm reduction has received impetus over the past decade because of the spread of AIDS: drug use is one of the risk behaviors most frequently associated with human immunodeficiency virus (HIV, or the virus thought to be necessary for AIDS). In some areas, IDU has become the main route of drug administration, and globally, it is now one of the primary risk factors for HIV infection. For example, in the United States, more than 20% of reported AIDS cases are directly associated with a history of injecting, and more than 30% of new HIV infections are in injection drug users. In some areas of Europe, injection of drugs accounts for as many as 60% of AIDS cases. What is more significant still is the rate at which HIV can spread among injection drug users. In cities such as Barcelona, Edinburgh, Milan, and New York, between 50% and 60% of drug users have become infected. In Thailand, where less than 1% of users were infected in January 1988, more than 40% were positive by September of that year, with a monthly incidence rate of 4% (Rana, 1996). Less than a decade later in the north-eastern province of Chiang Rai, one in six male military recruits and one in eight pregnant women were infected with HIV (Rana, 1996).

In all countries, HIV infection is not just a concern for the drug users themselves but also for their sexual partners. A number of studies in the United States and the United Kingdom have shown that between 60% and 100% of heterosexually acquired HIV is related to IDU, and that at least 40% of IDUs are in relationships with nonusers (Drucker, 1986; Rhodes, Myers, Bueno, Millson, & Hunter, 1998). Because of sexual spreading from injection drug-using partners, and because approximately one third of IDUs are female, vertical spreading to newborn children occurs. The possibility of transmission to the noninjecting community is increased by the fact that prostitution is sometimes used as a means of obtaining money for drugs, and many prostitutes are regular or occasional injectors. In addition, IDUs are a potential source of perinatal transmission: more than 50% of all pediatric AIDS cases in the United States are associated with injection drug use by one or both parents.

AIDS has thus been a catalyst for the rise in popularity of harm reduction. Before the AIDS pandemic, drug use was associated with a relatively low mortality rate because of periods of abstinence and natural recovery (Brettle, 1991; Wille, 1983). During the 1980s, there was a rapid increase in both AIDS and non-AIDS-related deaths in drug users (Stroneburneretal, 1989). Brettle (1991) has suggested that "this increase in mortality for drug users is the driving force behind harm reduction and the reason we can no longer rely on spontaneous recovery for drug users" (p. 125). This is no doubt a correct assessment of the primary force behind harm reduction, but it is by no means a full account of it. In North America in particular, harm reduction attracted attention because of the effects of drug prohibition other than the spread of AIDS alone. The violent crime, gang warfare, prison overcrowding, and police corruption associated with prohibition have reached a level such that policymakers, practitioners, and members of the public alike are seeking alternatives to prohibitionist drug policy.

It has been claimed that attempts to legislate and enforce abstinence are counter productive, and that there are harms due to these measures that are far worse than the effects of the drugs themselves (Erickson, 1992; Nadelmann, 1993; O'Hare, 1992; Riley & Oscapella, 1997). The harm reduction approach attempts to identify, measure, and minimize the adverse consequences of drug use at a number of levels, not just that of society as a whole. In a harm reduction framework, the term risk is used to describe the probability of drug-taking behavior resulting in any of a number of consequences (Newcombe, 1992). The terms harm and benefit are used to describe whether a particular consequence is viewed as positive or negative. In most cases, drug-taking behaviors result in several kinds of effects: beneficial, neutral, and harmful. The consequences of drug use can be conceptualized as being of three main types: health (physical and psychological), social, and economic. These consequences can be said to occur at three levels: individual; community (family, friends, colleagues, etc.); and societal (the structures and functions of society). They can also be broken down with respect to the time of their occurrence, into short-term and long-term effects. It is clear, given the wide range of moral and political views on the subject, that some consequences of drug use will remain highly controversial, and that assigning a positive or negative value will be purely subjective. Nevertheless, the harm reduction framework can be used as a means of better objectifying the evaluation process with respect to both drug programs and policies by allowing for the identification of harms that are to be dealt with.

The roots of harm reduction are in the United Kingdom, the Netherlands, and North America (Riley, 1993, 1994). Merseyside became a center for harm reduction policy because, like many other areas of the United Kingdom, it witnessed an epidemic spread of drug use, particularly heroin, in the early 1980s. Three important factors led to the establishment of the Mersey model of harm reduction. The first was the policy of the local drug dependency clinic, which was based on the old British system. Merseyside's major city, Liverpool, did not have its own drug dependency clinic until the mid-1980s. Prior to this, outpatient drug treatment was limited to a few psychiatrists who, in contrast to doctors in most other parts of the country, did not completely abandon the old British system. The British system emerged as a response to the recommendations of the Rolleston Committee, a group of leading physicians, on treatment of drug abusers in England during the 1920s. One of the most significant conclusions of the committee was that in certain cases, maintenance on drugs may be necessary for the patient to lead a useful life. To this day, injectable opiates have continued to be prescribed on a take-home basis in Merseyside.

A second factor in the emergence of the Mersey model was that in 1986, the Mersey Regional Drug Training and Information Centre began one of the first syringe exchange schemes in the United Kingdom, with the aim of increasing the availability of sterile injecting equipment to drug users in the area. The third factor was the cooperation of the local police, who agreed not to place drug services under observation and began to refer to drug services those drug users who had been arrested, a policy known as "cautioning."

In Merseyside, the harm reduction services include needle exchange; counseling; prescription of drugs, including heroin; and employment and housing services. One of the reasons that the Merseyside approach has proven so effective is that many levels of service and a wide variety of agencies are involved. The services for the drug user are integrated so that they can obtain help more readily when they need it. Together, Mersey Authority and the Merseyside Police have devised a comprehensive and effective harm reduction strategy, which came to be known as the "Mersey Model" of harm reduction (O'Hare, 1992).

All of the available evidence on HIV infection among IDUs in Merseyside suggests that the Mersey HIV prevention strategy for IDUs is very effective (see Stimson, 1997, for a review of approaches to HIV among drug users in the United Kingdom). Contacts with drug users have increased steadily over the past 5 years, and anecdotal evidence suggests that the number of drug-related health problems seen by services has dropped. Self-reported sharing of injecting equipment has declined, indicating positive behavioral change. By the end of 1994, only 29 drug injectors were known to be HIV positive and resident in the region. Official statistics indicate a decrease in drug-related acquisitive crime in many parts of the region, whereas the national rate is increasing (HIT, 1996). It is thought that the low prevalence of crime and HIV infection can be related to the various policies for dealing with drug use in the area.

In the early 1980s, Amsterdam recognized that drug use is a complex, recurring behavior, and that reduction of harm means providing medical and social care while waiting for natural recovery in order to avoid some of the more harmful consequences of injection drug use (Buning, 1990). Needle exchange began in 1984 after the Junkie Union advocated and then initiated the first exchange in order to prevent the spread of hepatitis B among users (Buning et al., 1986; Buning, van Brussel, & van Santen, 1988). Amsterdam has taken a pragmatic and nonmoralistic attitude toward drugs, and this has resulted in a multifaceted system that offers a variety of harm reduction programs. Police in the Netherlands focus attention and resources on drug traffickers, not users.

Although North America is not usually thought of in connection with harm reduction, Canada and the United States have been home to a very significant harm reduction strategy. One of the earliest forms of harm reduction for IDUs were methadone maintenance programs that began in Canada in the late 1950s and in the United States in the early 1960s. Methadone maintenance was seen as harm reduction for society, usually in terms of the reduction of crime or the reentry of drug users to the workforce (Brettle, 1991); improvement of the individual's physical health or protection of their human rights was not a priority. The spread of AIDS in opiate users has changed the entry and evaluation criteria for methadone programs, and it has also highlighted the need to modify these programs in order to reduce individual as well as societal harms (Jurgens & Riley, 1997; Newman, 1987; Springer, 1990).

A number of countries and organizations have now adopted harm reduction as both policy and practice. For example, the British Advisory Council on the Misuse of Drugs (1988) responded to the spread of HIV in IDUs by revising its policy on drug use to one of harm reduction: "We have no hesitation in concluding that the spread of HIV is a greater danger to individual and public health than drug misuse. Accordingly, services which aim to minimize HIV risk behaviour by all available means should take precedence in developmental plans" (para. 2.1). The World Health Organization (1986) has expressed a similar opinion, stating that policies aimed at reduction of drug use must not be allowed to compromise measures against the spread of AIDS.

THE NATURE OF HARM REDUCTION

Features of Harm Reduction

The essence of harm reduction is embodied in the following statement: "If a person is not willing to give up his or her drug use, we should assist them in reducing harm to himself or herself and others" (Buning, 1993, p. 1). The main characteristics or principles of harm reduction are as follows:

Pragmatism. Harm reduction accepts that some use of mind-altering substances is inevitable, and that some level of drug use is normal in a society. It acknowledges that, although carrying risks, drug use also provides the user with benefits that must be taken into account if drug-using behavior is to be understood. From a community perspective, containment and amelioration of drug-related harms may be a more pragmatic or feasible option than efforts to eliminate drug use entirely.

Humanistic values. The drug user's decision to use drugs is accepted as fact, as his or her choice; no moralistic judgment is made to either condemn or support the use of drugs, regardless of level of use or mode of intake. The dignity and rights of the drug user are respected.

Focus on harms. The fact or extent of a person's drug use per se is of secondary importance to the risk of harms consequent to use. The harms addressed can be related to health, social, economic, or a multitude of other factors, affecting the individual, the community, and society as a whole. Therefore, the first priority is to decrease the negative consequences of drug use to the user and to others, as opposed to focusing on decreasing the drug use itself. Harm reduction neither excludes nor presumes the long-term treatment goal of abstinence. In some cases, reduction of level of use may be one of the most effective forms of harm reduction. In others, alteration to the mode of use may be more effective.

Balancing costs and benefits. Some pragmatic process of identifying, measuring, and assessing the relative importance of drug-related problems, their associated harms, and costs/benefits of intervention is carried out in order to focus resources on priority issues. The framework of analysis extends beyond the immediate interests of users to include broader community and societal interests. Because of this "rational" approach, harm reduction approaches theoretically lend themselves to systematic evaluation to measure their impact on the reduction of harms in both the short and the long term, thereby determining whether their cost is warranted compared to some other, or no, intervention. In practice, however, such evaluations are complicated because of the number of variables to be examined in both the short and long term.

Hierarchy of goals. Most harm reduction programs have a hierarchy of goals, with the immediate focus on proactively engaging individuals, target groups, and communities to address their most pressing needs. Achieving the most immediate and realistic goals is usually viewed as the first step toward risk-free use, or, if appropriate, abstinence (e.g., see the guidelines from the Advisory Council on the Misuse of Drugs).

DEFINITION

At present, there is no agreement in the addictions literature or among practitioners as to the definition of harm reduction. One working definition is the following: "an attempt to ameliorate the adverse health, social or economic consequences of mood-altering substances without necessarily requiring a reduction in the consumption of these substances" (Heather, Wodak, Nadelmann, & O'Hare,1993, p. vi).

In the literature, the term harm reduction is often used interchangeably with the lesser-used term harm minimization. Two additional terms that are frequently used synonymously with harm reduction are risk reduction and risk minimization. Other terms occasionally used in conjunction with harm reduction are responsible drug use, problem prevention, secondary prevention, and risk management.

The definition of harm reduction has become an issue because of the broad nature of the term, its multiple meanings, and the conceptual fuzziness of the area in general. This has led to confusion among both harm reduction practitioners and its critics. For example, imprisonment of drug users for simple possession is, at present, construed by some to be a form of harm reduction. Practitioners dedicated to abstinence may also think of themselves as reducing the harms of substance abuse.

Harm reduction can be viewed as both a goal-the reduction of the number of harms associated with drug use-and a strategy-a specific approach that focuses on the negative consequences of drug use rather than on level of use. In both cases, one of the key definitional points is that the person's use of drugs is accepted as fact. Harm reduction approaches, then, are those that aim to reduce the negative consequences of drug use for the individual, the community, and society while allowing that a person may choose to continue to use drugs. This does not mean that harm reduction approaches preclude abstinence, only that there is acceptance of the fact that there are many possible approaches or strategies that can be taken to address drug-related problems, harm reduction and abstention being two of these. A harm reduction approach to a person's drug use in the short term does not rule out abstinence in the longer term, and vice versa.

Amid these diverse applications and levels of generality, the unique meaning and value of harm reduction as a concept and programming approach can easily be lost. This argues for a more restrictive definition of harm reduction, such as the following: "A policy or program directed toward decreasing adverse health, social, and economic consequences of drug use while the user continues to use drugs."

UNDERSTANDING "HARMS"

On the surface, it is easy enough to understand and endorse the primary goal of reducing the harms associated with drug use. Beyond that, however, it can be very difficult to get a clear picture of what exactly constitutes a harm, and to whom. The literature describes a broad range of harms. Most are attributed directly to drugs and behaviors related to their use; other harms are seen as resulting from the policies and programs in place to deter drug use. Thus, questions such as: What constitutes a harm as opposed to a benefit? To whom? What harms should be given priority, and when? can become very difficult to answer in practice.

Another area of debate concerns whether or not dependence constitutes a harm in and of itself. Consistent with the principles of harm reduction, many of its proponents do not view dependence as the priority; rather, they aim at reducing the clearly harmful consequences associated with drug use without requiring elimination of use itself. Practitioners of solely abstinence-oriented programs often view this as an unacceptable aspect of harm reduction.

Harm reduction takes a rational approach to drugs and requires a framework for identifying and assessing the relative effects of various kinds of drug use. This, in turn, rests on some classification of effects; some methodology for counting and costing the negative and positive outcomes of drug use; and a database from which to make comparative assessments of drug-related consequences for different types of drugs, target groups, and settings. In the majority of countries the elements of such a framework exist in fragmented form only. In the absence of objective data, much of the planning and delivery of harm reduction programs to date has been based on observation of risks and perceived priority of interventions.

RELATIONSHIP TO OTHER APPROACHES

Despite the current prominence of harm reduction, the notion of reducing harms associated with drug use has a long history. It has been a feature of British drug policy in particular for many decades, periodically surfacing and then fading (Berridge, 1993). This idea is firmly rooted in public health practice to secondary prevention with high-risk groups. Thus, harm reduction is neither a new nor an alternative approach so much as it is an extension and focusing of existing and accepted approaches.

Many harm reduction-based programs, such as needle exchanges, are of recent origin. Others, however, have a long and proven history; methadone programs, for example, date back to the 1960s and have demonstrated their effectiveness in assisting drug users to stabilize and normalize their lifestyles and in providing many with a bridge to abstinence from narcotic use. Helping people avoid harms has also been an established part of the alcohol field for many years; examples include promotion of responsible drinking, controlled drinking interventions, avoidance of drinking and driving, and low-alcohol-content beverages.

The recent increase in popularity of harm reduction is linked primarily to an increase in the influence of public health-based approaches to drug use and AIDS. Harm reduction is closely linked to a public health perspective through the sharing of common concepts and tools. In particular, harm reduction falls neatly in the conceptual framework of health promotion, with the minimization of risks and harms forming one part of the broader continuum of strategies to promote health and avoid disease. Both approaches emphasize the importance of respecting individuals and empowering them to increase opportunities to maximize their health, whatever the circumstances. As such, harm reduction, like health promotion, fits well with approaches that emphasize the importance of understanding the broad determinants of health and ensuring cost-effective approaches to the well-being of the entire population.

With respect to legal approaches, harm reduction in and of itself does not favor any one regulatory system over another. Rather, the issue is seen as an empirical one to be addressed through determining how best to regulate drugs in order to achieve a balance in minimizing harms to the individual, the community, and society as a whole. Nevertheless, advocates of harm reduction have been criticized severely for this view, with some opponents in North America, in particular, arguing that harm reduction is tantamount to advocacy for drug legalization. Although they do not necessarily favor legalization, many harm reductionists do believe that policies of drug prohibition have served only to exacerbate drug-related harm (Hawks, 1993; Jurgens & Riley, 1997; Kirby, 1996; Lurie & Drucker, 1997; Nadelmann, 1993; Riley & Oscapella, 1997).

THE PRACTICE OF HARM REDUCTION

Harm Reduction Programs and Policies
Syringe Exchange and Availability

Needle and syringe exchange programs are, to many people, the epitome of the harm reduction approach. They were first established in a few European countries in the mid- 1980s and, by the end of the decade, were operating in numerous cities around the world. The rationale behind syringe exchanges is that many people who are currently injecting are unable or unwilling to stop, and intervention strategies must help reduce their risk of HIV infection and transmission to others. Provision of sterile needles and syringes is a simple, inexpensive way to reduce the risk of spreading HIV infection. It is also a way of providing contact with drug users through outreach services. The strategy is based on a knowledge and means approach to behavioral change: People are provided with information about the changes that are needed and also with the means to bring about this change (sterile needles, syringes, other "works," and condoms).

Some exchange programs provide outreach services in the form of mobile vans or street workers to deliver services to drug scenes or to users' homes. Automated syringe exchange machines are now being used in many European and Australian cities. These vending machines release a clean syringe when a used one is deposited. Such machines are fairly inexpensive and accessible on a 24-hour basis. The machines, however, decrease the important personal contact between drug users and health care workers. In Amsterdam, which has the world's oldest syringe exchange (1984), and where there is a broad range of out-reach services to hard-core drug users, even some police stations will provide clean syringes on an exchange basis to people detained or arrested.

In areas where syringes cannot be made available, bleach kits (containing bleach and instructions for cleaning equipment) can be distributed. Although bleach is not totally effective in eliminating HIV and does not kill the pathogen that causes hepatitis (CDC, 1993), such kits help to reduce the likelihood of infection being passed through sharing of dirty equipment.

There is now clear direct and indirect evidence that attendance at syringe exchanges and increased syringe availability are associated with a decrease in risk (e.g., decreased sharing) as well as a decrease in harm (e.g., lower levels of HIV infection, increased access to medical care) (Hart, Carvell, Woodward et al., 1989; Jurgens, 1996; Lurie & Reingold, 1993; Rana, 1996; Robertson, 1990; Stimson, 1989, 1997; Stimson et al., 1988; van den Hoek, van Haastrecht, & Coutinho, 1989; Wodak, 1990, 1996).

Despite fears and propaganda to the contrary, needle exchanges are not associated with an increase in the number of injectors or a decrease in the average age of injectors. Thus, needle exchange has been shown to be a highly cost-effective means of reducing injection-related harms. In Australia, for example, early intervention with needle exchange programs and rapid tenfold expansion of methadone treatment kept the HIV rate among injection drug users below 2% after 1988 (Wodak, 1990, 1996).

The situation is markedly different in the United States, which has remained, for the most part, resistant to the adoption of harm reduction strategies. In 1996, Peter Lurie and Ernest Drucker used modeling techniques to estimate the number of HIV infections associated with the U.S. government's opposition to needle exchange programs. They estimated that between 4,000 and 10,000 IDUs in the United States would not now be infected with HIV had they had access to clean needles. Using the estimate of US$119,000 for the lifetime cost of treating an HIV infection, the authors conclude that these infections have cost the U.S. health care system some US$250 to US$500 million. The model does not include the indirect costs of HIV infection and uses conservative estimates. The median annual budget of a needle exchange in

North America is US$168,650. The average cost per syringe distributed is just US$1.35 (Lurie & Drucker, 1997). Two national AIDS commissions, the National Academy of Science's Institute of Medicine, and leading government experts have called repeatedly for repeal of the ban on needle exchange funding, but federal health authorities still maintain that harm reduction programs give the wrong message. The U.S. government, fearing that a move toward harm reduction will be viewed as a softening of its stance on illicit drugs, remains committed to prohibition and all of the many harms, including death, that attend it,

An important new development is the operation of needle exchange programs in an increasing number of prisons, primarily in Switzerland (Jurgens, 1996; Jurgens & Riley, 1997). Syringe exchange helps to prevent the spread of HIV and hepatitis in prisons and to fulfill legal and ethical obligations toward inmates, staff, and the public. Following their success in several prisons in Switzerland, programs to provide sterile needles have started in Spain and Germany (Jurgens, 1996). The Swiss found that the health status of prisoners improved, no new cases of infection with HIV or hepatitis occurred, a decrease in needle sharing was observed, there was no increase in drug consumption, and needles were not used as weapons. Several other countries, including Australia and Canada, are currently studying the feasibility of providing syringe exchange in their correctional facilities.

METHADONE PROGRAMS

Although methadone programs began in Canada and the United States, many of these programs have been criticized for their failure to provide the flexibility and range of services necessary for a cost-effective, harm-reducing program (Riley, 1993, 1995; Springer, 1990). Methods of providing methadone in the United Kingdom, the Netherlands, and Australia offer some examples of the range of possibilities necessary for effective harm reduction.

In the Netherlands, methadone is used in three different ways-to contact, stabilize, and detoxify/treat heroin users. By providing methadone without too many impediments – "low-threshold programs" – contact can be made with large sections of the heroin-using population. For example, there is a methadone bus program in which buses are used to distribute methadone throughout the drug-using community (no take-home dosages are provided). The primary disadvantages of the Dutch programs appear to be that they, like the U.S. programs, do not maintain all clients on levels of methadone that are high enough to prevent use of heroin, and they do not provide anything other than oral methadone.

Measures introduced to combat the spread of AIDS in Australia included the marked expansion of methadone programs. The criteria for admission to these programs were also made less stringent, and many more spaces were allowed for maintenance of clients with little motivation to change drug-using behavior. These changes to drug programs have been supported by a change in national and state policy toward drug abuse such that the highest priority has been given to the containment of HIV.

In the United Kingdom, parts of continental Europe, and Australia, methadone is available from clinics as well as general practitioners, who provide health care and counseling. In a number of European cities, more than 25% of all general practitioners prescribe methadone. Users pick up their prescription from pharmacies. Amsterdam, Barcelona, Frankfurt, and other cities distribute methadone through methadone buses or mobile clinics. Opiate-substitute programs in Canada are, at present, very limited both in terms of size and in terms of the options available to users (Riley, 1996).

There have been numerous studies on the effectiveness of methadone, and the vast majority of these have shown that methadone reduces morbidity and mortality, reduces the users' involvement in crime, curbs the spread of HIV, and helps drug users to gain control of their lives (Ball & Ross, 1991; Dole, 1989; Fazey, 1992; Gossop, 1978; Newman, 1976, 1987; Rana, 1996; Wodak, 1990, 1996; WHO, 1989, 1990). In all countries, one of the key factors underlying the success of methadone as a harm reduction measure is that it brings the user back into the community rather than treating him or her like an outsider or a criminal. This not only allows for rehabilitation of the user but it also means that the drugs and crime cycle can be broken. The experience of other countries shows that methadone programs work best if they are numerous, accessible, flexible, and liberal. Such expansion should take into account the need for methadone programs in prisons as well as the advantages of offering methadone treatment as an alternative to imprisonment and other forms of criminalization.

In prison itself, methadone programs are usually not available, creating problems and health risks for prisoners who were on methadone on the outside. A small but increasing number of prison systems worldwide are offering methadone maintenance to inmates, and a study undertaken in Australia suggests that the reduction of injecting and syringe sharing demonstrated in methadone programs in community settings also occurs in prisons (see Jurgens, 1996, for a review). A recent court case in British Columbia, Canada, may mean that methadone will be made available to some prisoners in that province. Currently, because many drug users end up spending time in prisons, it is important to ensure wider availability of methadone in prisons, and to explore the advantages of offering methadone treatment as an alternative to imprisonment.

PRESCRIBING OF DRUGS OTHER THAN METHADONE

In a tradition dating back to the 1920s, physicians in the United Kingdom prescribe drugs to users. In many regions, these services are provided through drug dependency clinics or community drug teams. These services offer flexible prescribing regimes ranging from short-term detoxification to long-term maintenance. The majority of clients receive oral methadone, but some receive injectable methadone; others receive injectable heroin; and a small number receive amphetamines, cocaine, or other drugs. These drugs are dispensed through local pharmacists (HIT, 1996; O'Hare, 1992; Riley, 1993, 1994).

In some parts of the United Kingdom, users can also be prescribed smokable drugs in the form of reefers. Drug users who are able to give up injecting often find that they are not able to switch immediately to oral prescriptions that do not provide the "rush" that an injected drug does (Palombella, 1990; Riley, 1993). Smokable drugs do provide a rush, although less powerful. In the Mersey region, where prescribing and other harm reduction programs are well established, anecdotal evidence suggests that drug-related health problems seen by services and acquisitive crime have decreased as a result of these services. There is a relatively high prevalence of heroin use, with there being an estimated 15,000 regular heroin users, of whom at least 50% inject. In 1994, the Mersey region had the second highest rate of notified addicts (4,088) of any regional health authority in the UK. The level of HTV infection among drug injectors in the Mersey region is very low (HIT, 1996).

Switzerland is carrying out a national experiment with prescribing of heroin and other drugs to users. The experiment is being conducted to determine whether prescribing of heroin and other drugs legally to users will reduce the users' criminal activity and their risk of contracting and spreading AIDS and other infections. The Swiss studied the British prescribing programs before setting out on the largest and most scientific study of heroin maintenance ever attempted. The program started in January 1994 with sites in eight cities. In each city, the program offers accommodation, employment assistance, treatment for disease and psychological problems, clean syringes, and counseling. Users are in regular contact with health workers and links to drug-free treatment. Some programs started off by giving some users heroin and others morphine or injectable methadone. It was soon found, however, that most users preferred heroin, which is provided up to three times a day for a small daily fee. Two programs allow clients to take a few heroin reefers home each night. Preliminary reports on the program suggest that heroin maintenance is efficacious (there were insufficient data to draw conclusions about cocaine). The programs have not resulted in a black market of diverted heroin, and the health of the addicts in the programs has clearly improved. The authorities have concluded from these preliminary data that heroin causes very few, if any, problems when it is used in a controlled manner and is administered under hygienic conditions. Based on these findings, the Swiss government expanded the program to more than 1,000 users in 1995 (approximately 800 slots for heroin, 100 each for morphine and injectable methadone) (Haemig, 1997). As part of this program, eight inmates in one prison in Switzerland are being maintained on heroin, so far with good results.

Holland began a heroin maintenance experiment in 1997, and several German cities would also like to begin programs. The Australian Capital Territory is also preparing to institute a heroin maintenance program.

EDUCATION AND OUTREACH PROGRAMS

Educational materials about drugs that have a harm reduction focus are readily available in a number of countries, including the United Kingdom, Holland, and Australia, but they remain extremely controversial and are often unavailable in most other countries. Although not promoting drug use, such materials tell the user how to reduce the risks associated with using drugs, teaching such things as safer injecting practices. In some countries, such as the United Kingdom, these techniques are taught by nurses at clinics.

In many countries, outreach workers are used to contact people such as drug injectors and prostitutes at risk of becoming infected with HIV. These workers distribute educational material, syringes, condoms, and bleach kits, and they help users contact other services.

LAW ENFORCEMENT POLICIES

Merseyside police in the northwest of England have devised a harm reduction approach known as "responsible demand enforcement" (Merseyside Police Force, 1990; Riley, 1993, 1994). They developed a cooperative harm reduction strategy with the regional health authority to improve the prevention and treatment of drug problems, particularly with respect to the spread of HIV infection among IDUs. The police are represented on Health Authority Drug Advisory Committees and employ health authority officers on police training courses involving the drugs/HIV issue. They have also supported the health authority by agreeing not to conduct surveillance on them, referring arrested drug offenders to services, not prosecuting for possession of syringes that are to be exchanged, and publicly supporting syringe exchange. One of the most important features of the Merseyside police strategy has been its emphasis on using resources to deal with drug traffickers while operating a cautioning policy toward drug users. Cautioning, which has now been adopted to some extent by all police authorities in Great Britain, has been recommended by the Attorney General of the United Kingdom as an appropriate option for some classes of offense, such as drug possession. Cautioning involves taking an offender to a police station, confiscating the drug, recording the incident, and formally warning the offender that any further unlawful possession of drugs will result in prosecution in court. The offender must also meet certain conditions, such as not having a previous drug conviction and not having an extensive criminal record. The offender is also given information about treatment services in the area, including syringe exchanges. The first time an offender is cautioned, he or she is not given a criminal record. On the second and third occasions, the offender is sent to court, where he or she is fined for possession of small quantities and sentenced for possession of large amounts. If an addict becomes registered through getting in touch with service agencies, then he or she is legally entitled to carry drugs prescribed to them for personal use. The overall effect of this policy is to steer users away from crime and possible imprisonment. In recent years, the approach has been extended to ecstasy, amphetamine, and cocaine, as well as heroin. In Merseyside, approximately 50% of drug possession incidents are dealt with by cautioning; in the rest of the United Kingdom, this figure is 25% (Dorn, personal communication, 1996).

In the Netherlands, police have long been supportive of harm reduction programs, including de facto decriminalization of marijuana and tolerance zones; enforcement efforts are concentrated on large-scale traffickers and on ensuring a safe and peaceful environment. As previously noted, some police stations in Amsterdam will provide clean syringes on an exchange basis. In Hamburg, Germany, a recent policy shift to harm reduction has been reflected in cooperation between police, health officials, and drug users' groups working together to help drug users access social services.

TOLERANCE AREAS

One innovative harm reduction approach being practiced in several European cities involves toleration by authorities of facilities known as "injection rooms," "health rooms," "contact centers," or similar terms. These are facilities where drug users can get together and obtain clean injection equipment, condoms, advice, medical attention, and so forth. The majority of these places allow users to remain anonymous. Some include space where drug users, including injectors, can take drugs in a comparatively safe environment. This is regarded as better than the open injection of illicit drugs in public places or consumption of drugs in "shooting galleries" that are usually unhygienic and controlled by drug dealers.

In Switzerland, the first drug rooms were established by private organizations in Bern and Basel in the late 1980s. By the end of 1993, there were eight such facilities, most operated by city officials. Several other cities in the German-speaking parts of Switzerland opened drug rooms in 1994. An evaluation of three of these facilities after their first year of operation showed that they had been effective in reducing the transmission of HIV and the risk of drug overdose (Nadelmann, 1995). Drug rooms are also provided by programs in Germany and Australia.

In the Netherlands, Rotterdam has also informally adopted a policy known as the "apartment dealer" arrangement. Following this policy, police and prosecutors refrain from arresting and prosecuting dealers who are living in apartments providing they do not cause problems for their neighbors. This approach is part of a "safe neighborhood" plan in which residents and police work together to keep neighborhoods clean, safe, and free of nuisances.

Not all tolerance zones have been successful. The first Swiss attempt at an open drug scene, "Needle Park" in Zurich, grew unmanageable and was closed in 1992. A second attempt also became uncontrollable and was closed in March 1995.

In Germany, open drug scenes emerged in Frankfurt during the 1970s and settled in two adjacent parks in the 1980s when police officials decided that their earlier attempts to suppress them had failed. Local authorities in Frankfurt established three crisis centers next to the drug scenes, provided a mobile ambulance to provide needle exchange services and medical help, offered first aid courses to users, and provided a separate bus for prostitutes. The police maintained their policy of apprehending dealers but initiated a new policy of tolerating an open scene within a clearly defined area of one of the parks. These activities were carried out along with efforts to draw users away from the drug scene by providing accommodations and treatment centers outside the city center. These efforts proved successful, and in 1992, the park drug scene was shut down. The policy has led to a significant reduction in the number of homeless drug users, drug-related crimes, and drug-related deaths in the city (Schneider, 1993,1996).

Toleration and regulation of open drug scenes and apartment dealers are forms of informal control similar to those used to regulate illegal prostitution, These controls are also compatible with the philosophy of community policing. In addition, local residents are chiefly concerned about the safety and peacefulness of their neighborhoods, not with drug use itself. Public health and social service workers find that it is easier to provide services when drug scenes are readily accessible and relatively static.

ALCOHOL PROGRAMS

Moderate drinking programs. One means of reducing the harms associated with alcohol is to teach people to consume alcohol in a moderate or sensible manner. A number of programs have been designed for problem drinkers. These programs are targeted toward people for whom drinking seriously interferes with life in such ways as disrupting close relationships, causing health concerns, and impairing driving.

Standard drink labels. One means of reducing drug-related harm is to provide consumers with factual information about what they are consuming so that they may better regulate their consumption. Standard-serving information involves stating the amount of ethyl alcohol in the container in relation to the amount of alcohol in a normal or standard serving. Normally, the size of the serving is chosen to correspond to the amounts of alcohol typically found in standard servings of regular-strength beer, wine, and spirits-which are often approximately equal. It has been suggested that providing standard-serving information would better enable drinkers and servers to avoid intoxication, enable drivers to be sure that they are below the legal blood alcohol level for driving, and assist anyone who wished to drink at levels defined as "low risk" by health experts. Standard-serving information in terms of grams of alcohol has been introduced in Australia. Standard unit information has already been introduced on a voluntary basis by Australian wine producers and a chain of grocery stores in the United Kingdom.

Server intervention programs. One way to reduce the harms associated with immoderate alcohol consumption is to train servers to recognize impairment and intervene to limit it in their patrons. Studies show that trained servers are less likely to serve someone who is underage or intoxicated. The success of server training has been due to the support of the hospitality industry and the focus on the drinking environment. To date, efforts to reduce impaired driving have focused on deterrence via criminal sanctions or educational measures aimed at individual drivers. Civil liability and server training, on the other hand, are directed at situations that give rise to impaired driving.

NICOTINE POLICIES AND PROGRAMS

Harm reduction approaches to nicotine products focus on reducing the harms to the user as well as to the inhaler of secondhand smoke. They include a wide range of approaches, from policies controlling smoking in public places to delivery of nicotine through gum, patches, inhalers, and smokeless cigarettes.

Workplace policies. Workplaces in many countries have now adopted policies restricting smoking either to designated areas within the building or to the outside. These policies have been associated with a decrease in smoking in the adult population. Because several other interventions have occurred in this time period (e.g., increased taxes, aggressive education campaigns), it is difficult to determine the role that workplace policies have played in changing smoking patterns. However, these policies are clearly related to decreasing numbers of complaints pertaining to the effects of secondhand smoke.

Smoking in public places. Like workplace policies, policies restricting smoking in public places such as restaurants and shopping plazas have been accompanied by decreased levels of smoking in the adult population. For the same reasons, it is difficult to determine the extent to which these changes are a response to the specific intervention or part of an overall pattern. The clearest effects of public policies are on decreasing exposure to secondhand smoke.

Nicotine gum. Chewing gum containing low levels of nicotine has become a popular means of reducing the harms of tobacco (by elimination of smoking) while avoiding some of the withdrawal symptoms associated with cessation of cigarette use.

Nicotine patch. Nicotine patches are adhesive pads that stick to the skin and release small amounts of nicotine into the bloodstream. They are intended to reduce the withdrawal symptoms that accompany smoking cessation. Research has demonstrated that users are most successful at quitting smoking and staying off cigarettes when the patch is accompanied by some form of counseling or behavior modification. The nicotine patch addresses the physical addiction to nicotine but does not deal with the psychological and behavioral aspects of smoking. Nevertheless, it is an important tool in assisting users to reduce and even eliminate smoking, thereby reducing nicotine-related harm substantially.

Nicotine inhalers. Still in the developmental stage, this delivery system offers the benefits of a clean delivery system but the problems of ensuring delivery of safe doses remain.

Smokeless cigarettes. A tar-free cigarette was developed by at least one tobacco manufacturer in the 1960s. The product was not released onto the market, however, because the company's lawyers advised that this would alert the public to the harms caused by regular cigarettes, thereby implicating the company with respect to any future legal suits. Interest in the production of smokeless cigarettes has been renewed by the acceptance of the relationship between tar and lung cancer by the public and the courts.

MARIJUANA POLICIES

Several countries or parts thereof, including the Netherlands, South Australia, and Germany, have introduced de facto decriminalization of small amounts of cannabis as a harm reduction strategy. The main reasons put forward for marijuana law reform to decriminalize personal use and cultivation include the following:

❖ Laws requiring court appearances are very expensive in terms of both money and human resources, and they place extremely heavy demands on the court system. Decriminalization for personal use frees up resources that can be directed toward detecting large-scale drug traffickers and money launderers.

❖ A criminal conviction for using or cultivating small amounts of marijuana in private is a consequence that is out of proportion to the seriousness of the offense; it leaves large numbers of people with criminal records who might otherwise never have a record but who will be affected for life by the stigma.

❖ By relying on criminal prosecution procedures to deal with small-scale marijuana offenses, the law may be contributing to the belief among many young people who have experimented with marijuana that the dangers of other illicit drugs have been overstated.

❖ The decriminalization of marijuana use will maintain a separation of drug markets so that small-scale users will have no need to come into contact with whole sale drug dealers.

❖ Existing marijuana laws cause more harm to the users than the drugs themselves through erosion of civil liberties, fines, and imprisonment.

❖ The existing laws allow corruption in law enforcement agencies.

❖ A prohibitionist approach leads to an increase in the use and price of the prohibited substance and creates a market that is devoid of controls, quality, standards, and accurate information.

In each of the cases where marijuana law reform has occurred, the final decision was based on the fact that tile costs associated with the existing system were seen to be too high by many segments of society, and too many people were seen as being adversely affected by the existing laws. In all of the cases where de facto decriminalization of marijuana has occurred, reduced financial and social costs were achieved without an increase in the risks to the community associated with drug use in general, Other, longer-term benefits have stemmed from the separation of high- and low-risk drug markets.

BARRIERS TO HARM REDUCTION

There are numerous barriers to both the policy and practice of harm reduction in many countries. One of the main barriers to the adoption of non prohibitionist policies is idealism. Adopting harm reduction means accepting that some harm is inevitable, whereas the zero tolerance approach of the United States is an example of a policy that, by definition, excludes all compromise (cf. Hawks, 1993). Canada, like the United States, has inherited the abstentionist morality where total abstinence is seen as the only acceptable goal of treatment for "abuse" of legal drugs and the only acceptable normal state with respect to illicit drugs. In North America, the drug war mentality has built additional serious barriers: any seeming support for drug users has been construed by some as support for drug use. Although realism and pragmatism of the harm reduction approach would view total elimination of harm as unlikely, to seek to reduce harm does not preclude the elimination of harm; idealism and harm reduction are not mutually exclusive.

Society's failure to accept drug use as a legitimate form of risk taking poses a significant barrier. Whereas societies tolerate and even encourage some forms of risk that are associated with much greater likelihood of harm than drug use (such as car racing, mountain climbing, and jet-skiing), harm reduction is viewed as promoting something that is necessarily bad and evil.

Another barrier is that of the relative ease of applying the different approaches. The supply reduction approach is the easiest to apply because in the current political climate, it has more support than does harm reduction.

Religious and other beliefs that hold that people should be punished for committing sins against morality stand in the way of harm reduction. AIDS and other drug-related harms are viewed as just deserts (as long as they are someone else's problem).

Another obstacle is an increasing distrust in paternalism and state control (cf. Hawks, 1993). More and more, the state is seen as having no role in controlling health except for that of providing information and leaving the rest to the individual. Objections to intervention of the state undermine some harm reduction efforts, such as the removal of alcohol tariff barriers in the European Economic Community and the General Agreement on Tariffs and Trade. Thus, harm reduction efforts are failing behind as economic issues become of greater concern and social and environmental programs take second place.

Legal barriers, such as paraphernalia and other drug laws, can stand in the way of harm reduction. In some cases, these barriers are more perceived than real. In such cases, rewriting of the relevant legislation to explicitly allow for syringe exchanges would make it easier for communities all over to open sites. In many other cases, however, the barriers of legislation are very real indeed: in Canada, for example, despite claims to have a harm reduction drug strategy, the primary mode of response to drug problems is still criminalization. To decrease this barrier to harm reduction, we need to change either the laws on drug use, or the enforcement of these laws, or both. Where current laws and policies do act as barriers, enabling strategies can sometimes be put into place that allow these barriers to be effectively overcome so that, for example, condoms or clean needles are still made available (see Tawil, Verster, & O'Reilly, 1995, for a review).

Another impediment is lack of public education regarding the nature and effects of drug policy. For example, one of the chief obstacles in setting up a syringe exchange is lack of public education on injection drug use and AIDS. Once the public is aware that syringe exchanges help to significantly reduce the spread of AIDS, they are much more supportive of them (although not in their own backyards).

The lack of treatment and other services for drug users in many countries stands in the way of significant progress in the area of harm reduction. This criticism is particularly true of our correctional systems. Until more user-friendly services are available, we are unlikely to be able to put harm reduction into practice, and we will continue to be hypocritical in our overall approach to drug users. To maximize contact with drug users, services can no longer afford to work only with those who seek to stop using drugs. It has been estimated that only 5% to 10% of the drug-using population is prepared to consider entering an abstinence-oriented program at any time. Clearly, we have to find ways to work with the other 90%.

With respect to prescribing drugs, it is indeed unfortunate that the kinds of prescribing options available in the United Kingdom are available in so very few countries. The majority of countries have said "no" to prescribing as a viable option, although the AIDS crisis is causing a number of them to reevaluate the situation.

CONCLUSION

The popularity of harm reduction on an international scale is evidenced by the increasing support for the International Conference on the Reduction of Drug Related Harm, now in its tenth year, and by the recent formation of the International Harm Reduction Association (IHRA). Despite the increase in popularity among workers in the field, many health and addiction agencies in North America and elsewhere remain ambivalent about harm reduction as it pertains to alcohol and other drugs. Some have positioned it closer to primary prevention and demand reduction, thus avoiding its more controversial applications.

Harm reduction raises some difficult questions, but it is evident that debating these questions openly is better than ignoring them, as has been done all too often in the past. Comprehensive harm reduction programs that are culturally sensitive are necessary; harm reduction must be multifaceted, not just a singular intervention.

The data regarding such drug-related consequences as AIDS make it clear that we need a long-term plan for harm reduction. Risk reduction is a social process; it is not something that public health officials can impose. An effective program must provide multiple means for behavior change and needs to be conducted on a long-term basis.

Although effective in reducing a number of the negative consequences associated with drug use, harm reduction has several limitations:

❖ The development and promotion of harm reduction strategies has to take into account the particular drug problem prevalent in a community, as well as the ethnic, socioeconomic, and legal characteristics of that community, or they will have limited applicability. For example, methadone maintenance programs are not applicable to stimulant problems. In these cases, other measures, such as ready access to clean equipment or distribution of stimulants in a noninjectable form, might be more effective.

❖ New interventions must be designed to reach all segments of the drug-using population. For example, at present, needle exchanges have had less success attracting young or female IDUs than older males. They are also less effective at reducing high-risk behavior in constituencies where greater legal restrictions apply.

❖ Harm reduction for injection drug use results in increased use of clean needles but not of condoms, and so, obviously, it cannot prevent sexual transmission of HIV (Stimson, 1997). In many communities around the world, the rate of increase in heterosexual AIDS has equaled or overtaken the rate for injection drug use-related AIDS.

❖ Harm reduction approaches are used mainly in the developed world. To be truly effective on a global level, they need to be applied in developing countries and to rich and poor alike.

As noted above, the most obvious question raised by the harm reduction approach is the meaning of the term harm itself. In deciding what constitutes harm, which are to be reduced, and in what order, scientific, political, moral, and other factors are obviously brought to bear. There are as many applications of harm reduction as there are harms to be reduced, but one person's harm may be another's benefit-and there's the rub. It would be all too easy for the harms that are selected for reduction to become only society's harms and not those of the individual and the community as well. Indeed, there are many who believe that sending drug users to jail is a form of harm reduction, We need to clarify the nature of the harm reduction approach sufficiently in order to prevent such arbitrary designation. At the same time, we must be careful that harm reduction does not get taken over by the temperance mentality, of which it is but in extension (why harm reduction and not benefit augmentation?). In so doing, we must be careful that the harms to be reduced are those that are truly relevant and not, as has happened all too often in the past, just those that are politically or morally correct. Harm reduction, in the final analysis, is concerned with ensuring the quality and integrity of human life in all of its wonderful, awful complexity. Harm reduction does not portray issues as polarities but sees them as they really are: somewhere in between. It is an approach that takes into account the continuum of drug use and the diversity of drugs, as well as of human needs. As such, there are no clear-cut answers or quick solutions. Harm reduction, then, is based on pragmatism, tolerance, and diversity. In short, it is both a product and a measure of our humanity. Harm reduction is as much about human rights as it is about the right to be human.

REFERENCES

Advisory Council on the Misuse of Drugs. (1988). AIDS and drug misuse (Part 1), London: HMSO.

Advisory Council on the Misuse of Drugs. (1989). AIDS andd drug misuse (Part 2). London: HMSO.

Ball, J. C., & Ross, A. (1991). *The effectiveness of methadone maintenance treatment*. New York: Springer-Verlag.

Berridge, V. (1993). Harm reduction and public health: An historical perspective. In N. Heather, A. Wodak, E. Nadelmann, & P. O'Hare (Eds,), *Psychoactive drugs and harm reduction: From faith to science* (pp. 55-64). London: Whurr.

Brettle,R.P.(1991).HIV and harm reduction for injection drug users. AIDS, 5, 125-136.

Buning, E. (1990). The role of harm reduction programmes in curbing the spread of HIV by drug injectors. In J. Strang & G. V. Stimson (Eds.), *AIDS and drug misuse* (pp. 153-161). London: Routledge.

Buning, E. (1993, March). Presentation made at St. Lawrence Forum on harm reduction, Toronto.

Buning, E., van Brussel, G. H., & van Santen, G. (1988). Amsterdam's drug policy and its implications for controlling needle sharing. In *Needle sharing among intravenous drug abusers: National and international perspectives* (NIDA Research Monograph 80, pp. 59-74). Rockville, MD: NIDA.

Buning, E., Coutinho, R. A., van Brussel, G. H., et al. (1986). Preventing AIDS in drug addicts in Amsterdam. Lancet, i, 1435.

Centers for Disease Control and Prevention. (1993, April 19). *HIV/AIDS Prevention Bulletin*. Atlanta, GA: Author.

Dole, V. P. (1989). Methadone treatment and the AIDS epidemic. *Journal of the American Medical Association*, 262, 1681-1682.

Drucker, E. (1986). AIDS and addiction in New York City. *American Journal of Drug and Alcohol Abuse*, 12, 165-181.

Erickson,P. (1992, Summer).Political pharmacology:Thinking about drugs. *Daedalus*, pp. 239-267.

Fazey, C. S. J. (1992). Heroin addiction, crime and treatment. In P. A. O'Hare, R. Newcombe, A. Mathews, E. C. Buning, & E. Drucker(Eds.), *The reduction of drug-related harm* (pp. 154-161). New York: Routledge.

Gossop,M. (1978).Review of the evidence for methadone maintenance as a treatment for narcotic addiction. *Lancet, i*, 812-815.

Haemig, R. (1997, March). *The Swiss heroin trials: The second intermediary report*. Paper presented at the Eighth International Conference on the Reduction of Drug Related Harm, Paris.

Hart, G. J., Carvell, A. L. M., Woodward, N., et al. (1989). Evaluation of needle exchanges in central London: Behaviour change and anti-HIV status over I year. *AIDS, 3*, 261-265.

Hawks, D. (1993). Impediments to the adoption of harm reduction policies. In N. Heather, A. Wodak, E. Nadelmann, & P. O'Hare (Eds.), *Psychoactive drugs and harm reduction: From faith to science* (pp. 93-102). London: Whurr.

Heather, N., Wodak, A., Nadelmann, E., & O'Hare, P. (Eds.). (1993). *Psychoactive drugs and harm reduction: From faith to science*. London: Whurr.

HIT. (1996). *Reducing drug related harm in the Mersey region*. Liverpool, UK: Author.

Jurgens, R. (1996). HIV/AIDS in prisons: Final report. Montreal: Canadian HIV/AIDS Legal Network and Canadian AIDS Society.

Jurgens, R., & Riley, D. (1997). Responding to AIDS and drug use in prisons in Canada. *International Journal of Drug Policy, 8*(1), 31-39.

Kirby, J. (1996, July). *Opening address*. The Harm Reduction Satellite to the XIth International Conference on AIDS, Vancouver, BC.

Lurie, P., & Drucker, E. (1997). An opportunity lost: HIV infections associated with the lack of a national needle-exchange program in the United States. *Lancet, 349*, 604-08.

Lurie, P., & Reingold, A. L. (Eds.). (1993). *The public health impact of needle exchange programs in the United States and abroad*. Berkeley: University of California Press.

Merseyside Police Force. (I 990). *Responsible demand enforcement: A summary*. Unpublished report. Liverpool, UK: Author.

Nadelmann, E. (1993). Progressive legalizers, progressive prohibitionists and the reduction of drug-related harm. In N. Heather, A. Wodak, E. Nadelmann, & P. O'Hare (Eds.), *Psychoactive drugs and harm reduction: From faith to science* (pp. 34-35). London: Whurr.

Nadlemann,E.(1995).Beyond needle park: The Swiss maintenance trial. *The Drug Policy Letter, 27*, 12-14.

Newcombe, R. (1992). The reduction of drug-related harm: A conceptual framework for theory, practice and research. In P. A. O'Hare, R. Newcombe, A. Matthews, E. C. Buning, & E. Drucker (Eds.), *The reduction of drug-related harm* (pp. 1-14). New York: Routledge.

Newman, R. G. (1976). Methadone maintenance: It ain't what it used to be. *British Journal of Addiction, 71,* 183-186.

Newman, R. G. (1987). Methadone treatment. *New England Journal of Medicine, 317,* 447-450.

O'Hare, P. A. (1992). Preface: A note on the concept of harm reduction. In P. A. O'Hare, R. Newcombe, A. Matthews, E. C. Buning, & E. Drucker (Eds.), *The reduction of drug-related harms.* New York; Routledge,

Palombella, A. (1990). Prescribing of smokeable drugs. *International Journal of Drug Policy, 1,* 3 1.

Rana, S. (1996). Harm reduction in Asia. *AHRN Newsletter, 1,* 4-6.

Rhodes, T., Myers, T., Bueno, R., Millson, R., & Hunter, G. (1998). Drug injecting and sexual safety. In G. Stimson, D. Des Jarlais, & A. B all (Eds.), *Drug injection and HIV infection* (pp. 130-148). London: University College London.

Riley, D. M. (1993). *The policy and practice of harm reduction.* Ottawa, Canada: CCSA.

Riley, D. M. (1994). *The harm reduction model.* Toronto: The Harm Reduction Network.

Riley, D. M. (1995). Methadone and HIV/AIDS. *Canadian HIV/AIDS Policy & Law Newsletter, 2,* 1-14.

Riley, D. M. (1996). Drug testing in prisons. *International Journal of Drug Policy, 6*(2), 106-111.

Riley, D. M., Sawka, E., Connley, P., Hewitt, D., Poulin, C., Room, R., Single, S., & Topp, J. (1999). Harm reduction: Concepts and practice. *Substance Use and Misuse 34*(l), 9-24.

Riley D.M.Oscapelia, E.(1997). Canada's new drug law: Some implications for HIV/AIDS prevention in Canada. *International Journal of Drug Policy, 7*(3), 180-182.

Robertson, J. R. (1990). The Edinburgh epidemic: A case study. In J, Strang & G. V. Stimson (Eds.), *AIDS and drug misuse* (pp. 95-107). London: Routledge.

Schneider, W. (1993). How my city charted a new drug policy course. *The Drug Policy Letter, 21,* 7-9.

Schneider, W. (1996, July). Presentation at the Harm Reduction Satellite of the XIth International Conference on AIDS, Vancouver, BC.

Springer, E. (1990). AIDS prevention with drug users supplanted by the war on drugs, or what happens when you don't use harm reduction models. *International Journal on Drug Policy, 2,* 18-21.

Stimson, G. V. (1989). Syringe exchange programs for injecting drug users. *AIDS, 3,* 253-260.

Stimson, G. V. (1997, March). *Harm reduction in practice: How the UK can avoid an epidemic of HIV infection in drug injectors.* Paper presented at the Eighth International Conference on the Reduction of Drug Related Harm, Paris.

Stimson, G. V., Alldritt, L., Dolan, K., et al. (1988). *Injecting equipment exchange schemes.* Final report. London: Monitoring Research Group, Goldsmiths' College.

Stroneburner, R. L., DesJarlais, D. C., Benezra, D., et al. (1989). A larger spectrum of severe HIV-1 related disease in intravenous drug users in New York City. *Science, 242,* 916-918.

Tawil, O., Verster, A., & O'Reilly, K. R. (I 995). Enabling approaches for HIV/AIDS prevention:Can we modify the environment and minimize the risk? *AIDS, 9,* 1299-1306,

Van den Hoek, J.A.R., van Haastrccht, H.J.A., & Coutinho, R.A.(1989).Risk reduction among intravenous drug users in Amsterdam under the influence of AIDS. *American Journal of Public Health, 79,* 1355-1357.

Wille, R. (1983). Processes of recovery from heroin dependence: Relationship to treatment, social change and drug use. *Drug Issues, 13,* 333-342.

Wodak, A. (1990). AIDS and injecting drug use in Australia: A case control study in policy development and implementation. In J. Strang & G. V. Stimson (Eds.), *AIDS and drug misuse* (pp. 132-14 1). London: Routledge.

Wodak, A. (1996, July). *Harm reduction works.* Paper presented at the Harm Reduction Satellite to the XIth International Conference on AIDS, Vancouver, BC.

World Health Organization. (1986). Consultation an AIDS among drug abusers. Stockholm: World Health Organization Regional Office for Europe.

World Health Organization. (1989). *The uses of methadone in the treatment and management of opioid dependence.* Geneva.

World Health Organization. (1990). *The content and structure of methadone treatment programs: A study in six countries.* Geneva.

The Interconnected Epidemics of Drug Dependency and AIDS[1]

by Larry Gostin

Executive Director, American Society of Law & Medicine

Adjunct Associate Professor of Health Law, Harvard University

The first question one has to ask is whether drug dependency and AIDS are at all inter-connected. If they are, is there any evidence that a consistent policy on drug use that prefers public health approach rather than the restrictive approach actually works? HIV/AIDS is not the first disease that makes us ask all these questions, malaria and hepatitis are another example. Needle sharing among drug users represents a highly effective method of transmission of blood-borne diseases. The governmental prohibitions and criminal measures often render public health efforts ineffective. These policies focus on punishing the "immoral" behavior, but do not lower rates of drug use and infections. The first goal should be to prevent the sharing of needles and other injection paraphernalia to ensure the use of sterile injection equipment and to provide treatment and rehabilitation. Educational efforts are important and prove to be extremely effective in reducing the sharing of the works. However, none of the existing preventive strategies will significantly impede the spread of HIV if standing alone.

A half-century ago the humanist Edward M. Brecher reported a mid-winter epidemic of malaria in Chicago, New York City, St. Paul, and San Francisco. The epidemic occurred despite the absence of a single live mosquito, a common carrier of the disease.

Drug-dependent people in these cities were sharing the needles and syringes they used to inject heroin. If the drug-dependent person were infected with malaria parasites, his or her needle-sharing partner ran the risk of acquiring the infection.[2] The epidemic increased the next summer when mosquitoes bit malaria-infected drug users and transmitted the infection to the wider public.

Brecher's report demonstrated, as early as 1940, that intravenous (IV) drug users could spread an infectious disease to their needle-sharing partners, and from the partner to other women, men, and children.[3] Indeed, needle sharing has proven to be an effective secondary mode of transmission for a diverse range of blood-borne and sexually transmitted diseases such as bacterial endocarditis,[4] syphilis,[5] hepatitis,[6] cellulites,[7] and soft-tissue infections.[8]

Needle sharing among drug-dependent people is fueling the modern human immunodeficiency virus (HIV) epidemic in a pattern strikingly similar to its role in spreading other needle borne infections. The transmission of HIV occurs when infected drug users self-administer heroin, cocaine,[9] amphetamines or other drugs through an injection into a vein, under the skin or into a muscle ("skin popping"). The needle, syringe and possibly the "cooker"[10] may contain small amounts of HIV-infected blood. To ensure that no trace of the drug remains in the syringe, the user often draws his blood into the syringe and reinjects it into his vein, a practice known as "booting." The "works" are then shared with another drug-dependent person who draws his own blood into the syringe, mixing it with the blood from his partner. Thus, the syringe and needle sharing results in a highly efficient method of transmitting an infection.[11]

The needle-borne HIV epidemic is a public health problem of broad dimensions. Intravenous drug users are the second largest risk group for HIV infection in the American population. Twenty-nine percent of all cases of AIDS reported to the U.S. Centers for Disease Control involve IV drug users.[12] The serological prevalence of HIV in the IV drug use community is higher still. Epidemiological studies in major urban areas, particularly New York, Northern New Jersey, and Connecticut, demonstrate HIV seroprevalence rates of fifty percent or more.[13] Moreover, HIV disease in drug-dependent populations is an epidemic that strikes disproportionately the urban poor, African Americans and Hispanics.[14] Ethnographic studies of this population describe it as "street drug abusers," the vast majority of whom is homeless, unemployed, or underemployed. Many also suffer from multiple physical dependencies on drugs and alcohol.[15] These studies point to the vulnerability of the drug-dependent population and its frequent inability to meet its own health care needs.

HIV among IV drug users is also the single most important source for the spread of the infection to non-risk groups. It is likely that if heterosexual transmission of HIV becomes self-sustaining, IV drug users will be the source of infection.[16] Nearly seventy-two percent of all heterosexual cases of AIDS reported in the United States involve persons who have had sexual contact with an IV drug user.[17] The connection between pediatric AIDS an IV drug use is even more striking. Seventy-nine percent of all children born infected with HIV have a mother who either was an IV drug user or had sexual relations with an IV drug user.[18]

Drug dependence and HIV are America's two most pressing epidemics,[19] interconnected by a cycle of urban poverty, physical dependence and a culture of sharing needles and syringes.[20] Extant political strategies to curb these interconnected epidemics involve two traditional approaches. The first-law enforcement and interdiction is designed to limit the supply of illicit drugs to the marketplace. This strategy is advanced by broad criminal sanctions against importing, selling, distributing, medically prescribing, or possessing illicit drugs or drug paraphernalia. The second strategy to combat the drug and HIV epidemics involves reducing the demand for illicit drugs. Education, counseling, and treatment (detoxification, maintenance, and rehabilitation) are all designed to reduce dependence on drugs, and are called demand-side policies. For those who cannot stop drug use, public health strategies seek to alter dangerous sharing behavior or to encourage the sterilization of works.

Supply-side and demand-side policies are often in conflict, and this conflict reduces the efficiency of the programs and thwarts the public health goals that underlie both types of policies. For example, counseling, education, and outreach programs designed to teach drug-dependent people safer ways to engage in unlawful behaviors appear to condone or even foster drug use. Drug users who follow public health advice and carry clean injection equipment or bleach to sterilize that equipment may provide law enforcement personnel with evidence of criminal behavior. Similarly ex-addicts hired by public health departments to distribute drug injection equipment in shooting galleries come close to aiding and abetting the commission of a crime. Finally, needle and syringe exchange programs require the distribution of equipment with the knowledge that it will be used to inject drugs. Such acts are specifically prohibited under present drug-paraphernalia statutes.

The conflict between supply-side and demand-side policies is also reflected in the relative funding that the federal government commits to law enforcement and public health. Less than two decades ago only 44.1% of the federal drug abuse budget went to activities related to interdiction, eradication and other law enforcement, with the remaining funds going to drug treatment, prevention, and education. By 1976 the proportion was still relatively even with 50.4% going to law enforcement. In the last decade, however, expenditures for law enforcement rose substantially to between 73% and 82% of the drug abuse budget.[21] The increase in the enforcement budget reflects the current government philosophy that strong supply-side efforts that emphasize the criminal and immoral aspects of drug use will yield health benefits for the public.

The uniting theme of this Article is that government should pursue a consistent policy on drug use that explicitly prefers therapeutic and public health goals to law enforcement goals when these two are in conflict.[22] Such a preference for therapeutic goals is needed because of the seriousness of the HIV epidemic and because the sweep of criminal prohibitions and government regulation often renders public health measures ineffective.[23] A preference for public health over law enforcement is justified on both conceptual and empirical grounds.[24] The *raison d' etre* of the supply-side policies is to protect the health of the user and of the public. Thus the human tragedy of the drug and HIV epidemics is not simply that people are acting unlawfully or immorally, but that drug dependency is destructive to a person's health and to the health of the community. The goal of supply-side policies should be to protect the health and safety of the individual and the community, not simply to punish "immoral, self-gratifying" behavior.

Thus, the measure of effectiveness of those policies should be whether they succeed in lowering rates of drug dependency and needle-borne transmission of infection. If supply-side policies fail this test, they defeat the very objective for which they were formulated and lose their validity.

The nation's law enforcement strategy to curb the drug dependency and HIV epidemics has not been successful. The rate of serious drug use and the needle-borne spread of HIV are both growing in ways that are profoundly detrimental to the health of the public.[25] The United States has not attempted a comprehensive public health approach to confront the dual epidemics of drugs and HIV, yet, as this Article will demonstrate, scientific studies show that public health policies will be effective in reducing the demand for drugs, the sharing of drug-injection equipment, and the overall risk of HIV infection. Consistent with these studies and with a focus on demand-side policies, this Article presents three strategies for controlling the spread of HIV in the drug-dependent population.

The first public health strategy is to prevent the sharing of drug-injection equipment. Sharing could be prevented through the creation or expansion of education, counseling, and outreach programs. Highly disparate HIV prevalence rates exist among IV drug populations in the United States and abroad. The risk of HIV transmission does not exist if drug-dependent people use and reuse their own needles and syringes. Accordingly, the first strategy for breaking the cycle of HIV infection among drug-dependent people is to prevent the sharing of works.

The second public health strategy is to ensure that drug-dependent people use sterile injection equipment. Drug-dependent people can obtain access to safe injection equipment by sterilizing it themselves, by purchasing it over the counter, or by receiving it without charge pursuant to a publicly sponsored program. Education and counseling designed to teach safer forms of behavior cannot be successful unless the drug-dependent person has access to sterile injection equipment. This Article will discuss strategies aimed at making the use of sterile equipment a realistic option for drug users.

The third public health strategy is to provide medical treatment and rehabilitation so that the drug user is no longer dependent on drugs or can satisfy the craving through lawful use of a prescribed drug such as methadone. However, formidable obstacles stand in the way of universal access to drug treatment. ese obstacles include inadequate resources for treatment facilities, the sometimes prohibitive cost of treatment for individuals, zoning laws, and methadone regulations. This Article will develop ideas for substantially increasing the role of the health care and criminal justice systems in the treatment of drug dependency.

None of these strategies, standing alone, will significantly impede the spread of HIV in the drug-dependent population. But the cumulative effect of education, counseling, and outreach to reduce sharing of works; of clean-needle programs to increase the use of sterile injection equipment; and of comprehensive medical treatment in specialized and mainstream health facilities to reduce dependence on drugs provides the best opportunity to impede the needle-borne HIV epidemic. The political justification for the sweeping changes in law, policy, and public funding needed to meet this health imperative is found in saving the lives and health dollars of the drug-dependent population, their sexual and needle-sharing partners, their children, and, ultimately, the general population. A public health policy not only would effect a fundamental reduction in the morbidity and mortality stemming from the HIV epidemic, but would also lessen the severity of future needle-borne epidemics, which, as history has already demonstrated, will occur.

EDUCATION ABOUT RISK AVOIDANCE PRACTICES: PUBLIC POLICIES DESIGNED TO REDUCE SHARING OF DRUG PARAPHERNALIA

The sharing of works is the most critical factor in the transmission of HIV in the IV drug use populations.[26] Works are usually shared out of practical necessity, but sometimes sharing of works occurs as part of the drug subculture, as a form of social bonding or camaraderie within the group.[27] Drug-dependent persons share works with sexual partners, members of a friendship group or other users in a "shooting gallery."[28] A shooting gallery is a place where a person can inject illicit drugs. Most galleries are located near a "copping" place where drugs can be purchased.[29] Needles are sometimes obtained "free" with the drug purchase;[30] others, kept by dealers for renting or lending to customers, are called "house works."[31] After the house works are used, they are then returned and used again by another customer. Needles and syringes may be used repeatedly in this way until they become clogged with blood, too dull to use, or break.[32] Most users in research studies report that they obtain their needles from street sellers and shooting galleries.[33] Shooting galleries and house works are particularly detrimental to the public health because they involve sharing needles beyond a small group of friends or sexual partners.

Current education programs have successfully disseminated basic information about how AIDS is transmitted.[34] However, a striking dissonance still exists between what IV drug users know and how they behave.[35] Even though many addicts know that sharing is a high-risk behavior, they continue to share works because drug-dependent people going through withdrawal are concerned primarily with a rapid injection of heroin or cocaine.[36] Possession of heroin itself may create a premature withdrawal and craving in a long-term addict through a form of classical conditioning.[37] Withdrawal is extremely unpleasant, and thus an addict will not stop to plan or consider the health consequences when he is in need of a fix. Research indicates that addicts will use whatever equipment is available when they are in withdrawal.[38] Users, however, cannot rely on dealers and shooting gallery proprietors as a safe source of sterile equipment, since these dealers and proprietors sometimes repackage contaminated needles and syringes and sell them as new.[39] Since sterile injection equipment is not readily available, education programs must teach drug users how to sterilize the needles and syringes by themselves.

Risk-reduction education must also be designed to overcome the ingrained behavior of needle sharing and to help form new patterns of behavior in the drug-dependent population. Although complete abstention from drug use is an admirable goal, for many it will never be achieved. If society truly desires to promote health and save lives among persons who continue to inject drugs, risk-reduction education is critically important.

A. Can Education Work?

Public and political opposition to risk-reduction programs are evident across the nation.[40] Opponents often argue that these programs are unlikely to be effective because of the inherent characteristics of the IV drug-using population: physiological dependence, illiteracy and lack of formal education.[41] Opponents of risk reduction also argue that drug users have a fundamental lack of concern about their health. Finally, opponents point to the difficulty of reaching a group engaged in a criminal enterprise that the dominant population regards with hostility.

Arguments that risk-reduction programs cannot be effective ignore relevant data.[42] Studies show that an overwhelming majority of users know and understand the behavior that puts them at risk for HIV infection.[43] More significantly, drug-dependent persons have shown a willingness to change socially ingrained activities — evidenced by greater use of sterile injection equipment, fewer needle-sharing partners, and less IV drug use-when provided with education and counseling and given the means to change their behavior.[44] As a result of risk-reduction programs, drug users are demanding that dealers and proprietors of shooting galleries provide sterile injection equipment.[45] They have also sought out public health department programs, such as bleach and sterile needle distribution, and drug treatment.[46] Thus, risk-reduction education has successfully disseminated important information to drug users. An education program aimed at teaching drug users needle sterilization techniques and at breaking down sharing behavior should be similarly successful.

NOTES

[1] Taken from Harvard Civil Rights-Civil Liberties Law Review 26 1990/91 pp. 114-124. Used with permission.

[2] Brecher, The Case of the Missing Mosquitoes, READER's DIC ,EST, Feb. 1941, at 56. Heroin dealers attempted to impede the needle-borne malaria epidemic by adding quinine to the heroin "bag" to kill the malaria parasites. Brecher, Needles and the Cotiscience of a Nation, I DRUG POL'Y LETTER 5-6 (1989). See also E. BRECHER, LICIT AND ILLICITDRUGS (1972).

[3] See Drugs and Edward Brecher, N.Y. Times, Apr. 25, 1989, at A28, col. 1.

[4] Inflammation of the endocardium, or lining membrane of the heart, is caused by the direct invasion of bacteria and leads to deformity of the valve leaflets. STEDMAN'S MEDICAL DICTIONARY, 510 (25th ed. 1990) [hereinafter STFDMAN'S].

[5] Syphilis is an acute and chronic infectious disease caused by Treponeina pollidlim (Spirochaeta pallida) and transmitted by direct contact, usually through sexual intercourse. The late stages of the disease are marked by

formation of gummas and cardiovascular andcentral nervous system lesions. STEDMAN'S, supra note 32, at 1544.

[6] Hepatitis is an inflammation of the liver. The viral h, type B form of hepatitis is caused by hepatitis B virus (HBV) (serum hepatitis virus). Necrosis of liver cells is characteristic, and jaundice is a common symptom., STEDMAN'S, supra note 32, at 704-05. Transmission of HBV sexually and through contaminated needles is the model often used for HIV. See Blumber & Fox, The Daedalus Effect: Changes in Ethical Questions Relating to Hepatitis B, 102 ANNALS INTERNAL MED. 390, 394 (1985).

[7] Cellulitis is the inflammation of cellular or connective tissue. STEDMAN'S, supra note 3, at 273.

[8] See NATIONAL RESEARCH COUNCIL, AIDS: SEXUAL BEHAVIOR AND INTRAVENOUS DRUG USE 189 (C. Turner, H. Miller & L. Moses eds. 1989) [hereinafter NATIONALRESEARCH COUNCIL REPORT].

[9] Cocaine affects the HIV epidemic in two significant ways. First, cocaine can be injected. Indeed, intravenous cocaine users have to inject more frequently than heroin users to achieve the same high, thus posing a greater risk of transmission of HIV. Cur rently, there is no chemical treatment for cocaine use comparable to methadone for heroin use. For a discussion of methadone maintenance programs, see infra notes 251-253 and accompanying text. See also NATIONAL INSTITUTE ON DRUG ABUSE, U.S. DEPARTMENT OF HEALTH AND HUMAN SERVICES, NIDA MONOGRAPH No. 88, MECHANISMS OF COCAINE ABUSE AND TOXICITY (1988) [hereinafter NIDA MONOGRAPH No. 88]. Second, the exchange of sex for cocaine, particularly in crack houses, is fanning the HIV epidemic. See Fullilove, Thompson, Bowser & Gross, Risk of sexually Transmitted Disease Among Black Adolescent Crack Users in Oakland and San Francisco, California 263 J.A.M.A. 851 (1990). The sexual highs, the payment of money, and the propensity of cocaine users to neglect safer sexual practices are all reasons for deep concern about the drug's impact the HIV epidemic.

[10] A cooker is a spoon or bottle cap used to dissolve the drug in water prior to injection.

[11] See Des Jarlais, Friedman & Strug, *AIDS and Needle Sharing Within the IV Drug Use Subculture*, in THE SOCIAL DIMENSIONS OF AIDS: METHODS AND THEORY 111 (D. Feldman & T. Johnson eds. 1986); Ginzburg, *Intravenous Drug Abusers and HIV Infection: A Consequence of Their Actions*, 14 LAW, MED. & HEALTH CARE 268 (1986); Stryker, *IV Drug Use and AIDS: Public Policy and Dirty Needles*, 14 J. HEALTH POL'Y, POL. & LAW 719 (1989).

[12] CENTERS FOR DISEASE CONTROL, HIV/AIDS SURVEILLANCE: U.S. CASES REPORTED THROUGH SEPTEMBER 1990, at 8 (1990) thereinafter CENTERS FOR DISEASE CONTROL, SEPT. 19901. Cumulative totals of reported AIDS cases show that 22% were IV drug users and 7% were IV drug users and had had homosexual contact. Indeed, a significant number of deaths of IV drug abusers may be attributable to HIV disease but are not reported as CDC-defined AIDS. These deaths may represent a spectrum of HIV-related disease that has not been identified through AIDS surveillance and has resulted

in a large underestimation of the impact of AIDS on IV drug users, African Americans and Hispanics. Stoneburner Des Jarlais, Benezra, Gorelkin, Sotheran, Friedman, Schultz, Marmor, Mildvan & Maslansky, A Larger Spectrum of Severe HIV-1-Related Disease in Intravenous Drug Users in New York City, 242 SCIENCE 916 (1988); see NATIONAL RESEARCH COUNCIL REPORT, Supra note 37, at 234-37.

[13] See Des Jarlais, Friedman & Stoneburner, HIV Infection and Intravenous Drug Use: Critical Issues in Transmission Dynamics, Infection Outcomes, and Prevention, 10 REV OF INFECTIOUS DISEASES 151 (1988); Des Jarlais, Wish, Friedman, Stoneburner, Yancovitz Mildvan, El-Sadri Brady & Cuadrado, Intravenous Drug Use and the Heterosexual Transmission of the Human Immunodeficiency Virus: Current Trends in New York City, 87 N.Y. ST. J. MED. 283 (1987); Robertson, Bucknell, Welsby, Roberts, Inglis, Peutherer & Brettle, Epidemic of AIDS Related Virus (HTLV-III/LAV) Infection Among Intravenious Drug Users, 292 BRIT. MED, J. 527, 529 (1986). Needle-borne transmission of HIV, moreover, is an international phenomenon with comparably high rates of AIDS and HIV infection among IV drug users in parts of Europe. Approximately 18% of reported cases of AIDS in Europe indicate IV drug use as a risk factor (3% of these cases also had homosexual contacts). The percentage of people with AIDS who are IV drug users is significantly higher tain countries. For example, in Italy and Spain, IV drug users account for 65% and 59% of adult cases of AIDS, respectively. WORLD HEALTH ORGANIZATION, PROGRESS REPORT No. 4, 8, GLOBAL PROGRAMME on AIDS (1988); see Angrarano, Pastore, Monno, Santantonio, Luchena & Schiraldi, Rapid Spread of HTLV-111 Infection Among Drug Addicts in Italy, 2 LANCET 1302 (1985).

[14] Over 43% of all cases of AIDS reported to the CDC involve African Americans (28%) or Hispanics (nearly 16%). CENTERS FOR DISEASE CONTROL, SEPT. 1990, supra note I 1, at 12; see also Des Jarlais & Fricdman, HIV Infection Among Persons Who Inject Illicit Drugs: Problems and Prospects, 1 J. ACQUIRED IMMUNE DEFICIENCY SYNDROME 267, 269 (1988) (higher HIV seroprevalence among ethnic minority drug users). The risk factors are related to behavior, but not race. "To label a pigment as a risk factor is to promote . . . racist notions that have hampered HIV research, thwarted access to care, and tainted educational efforts about HIV," Dawson, HIV in Intravenous Drug Users, 322 NEW NC,. J.MED. 632 (1990).

[15] Feldman & Biernacki, The Ethnography of Needle Sharing Among Intravenous Drug Users and Implications for Public Policies and Intervetition Strategies, in NATIONAL INSTITUTE ON DRUG ABUSE, U.S. DEPAIITMENT OF HEALTH AND HUMAN SERVICES, NIDA MONOGRAPH No. 80, NEEDLE SHARING AMONG INTRAVENOUS DRUG ABUSERS: NATIONAL AND INTERNATIONAL PERSPECTIVES 28 (1988) [hereinafter NIDA MONOGRAPH No. 80].

[16] NATIONAL RESEARCH COUNCIL REPORT, supra note 37, at 2186.

[17] CENTERS FOR DISEASE CONTROL 1990, supra note II, at 9. This figure exclude s females born outside the United States in Pattern II countries, where heterosexual transmission patterns are more evident. In New York City almost

90% of the heterosexual transmission cases of AIDS involve sexual relations with an IV drug user. Des Jarlais & Friedman, The Psychology of Preventing AIDS Among Intravenous Drug Users, 43 Am.PSYCHOLOGIST 865 (1988).
[18] CENTERS FOR DISEASE CONTROL, SEPT. 1990, supra note I 1, at 9. This figure excludes females born in Pattern 11 countries where heterosexual transmission patterns are more evident.
[19] See generally NATIONAL RESEARCH COUNCIL REPORT, supra note 37; REPORT OF THE PRESIDENTIAL COMMISSION ON THE HUMAN IMMUNODEFICIENCY VIRUS EPIDEMIC 94-104 (1988) [hereinafter REPORT OF THE PRESIDENTIAL COMMISSION]; Schuster, A Federal Agency Perspective on AIDS, 43 Am. PSYCHOLOCIST 846, 848 (1988).
[20] See Three Plagues, N.Y. Times, Feb. 23, 1989, at A22, Col. 1
[21] Brecher, Needles and the Conscience of a Nation, supra note 30, at 5-6; see infra notes 276-282 and accompanying text.
[22] Some European countries have explicitly affirmed the importance of public health over law enforcement as a strategy for confronting the needle-borne HIV epidemic. See Fox, Day & Klein, The Power of Professionalism: Policies for AIDS in Britain, Sweden, and the United States, 118 DAEDALUS 93 (1989).
[23] Supply-side policies appropriately criminalize the importation and sale of illicit drugs, but they go further to impose criminal sanctions on people who are physically dependent on drugs. To be sure, the Constitution prohibits the criminal law from penalizing a person for the status of drug dependency. Robinson v. California, 370 U.S. 660 (1962). But penalties for simple possession of drugs or even drug paraphernalia go as far as is constitutionally permissible to impose criminal sanctions on individuals as a direct result of their medical illness.
[24] See Gostin, An Alternative Public Health Vision for a National Drug Strategy: "Treatment Works", 28 U. Hous. L. REV. (forthcoming 1991).
[25] The decline in casual drug use is a notable achievement of efforts to reduce illicit drug use. NATIONAL INSTITUTE ON DRUG ABUSE, NATIONAL HOUSEHOLD SURVEY ON DRUG ABUSE: POPULATION ESTIMATES 1988 (1989). However, this reduction in casual drug use may reflect prevention and education efforts in schools and significant cultural changes rather than the effectiveness of current law enforcement techniques. Moreover, the decline in casual use is more than offset by a marked increase in drug dependency and regular use of highly addictive drugs such as cocaine. THE WHITE HOUSE, NATIONAL DRUG CONTROL STRATEGY 1 (1989).
[26] See, e.g., Becker & Joseph, AIDS and Behavioral Change to Reduce Risk: A Review, 78 Am. J. PUB. HEALTH 403 (1988); Chaisson, Moss, Onislii, Osmond & Carlson, Human Immunodeficiency Virus Infection in Heterosexual Intravenous Drug Users in San Francisco, 77 Am. J. Pui3. HEALTH 169 (1987); Schoenbaum, Hartel, Selwyn, Klein, Davenny, Rogers, Feiner & Friedman, Risk Factors for Human Immunodeficiency Virus Infection in Intravenous Drug Users, 321 NEw ENO. J. MED. 874 (1989). For a useful description of the social context of needle sharing, including friendship networks and shooting galleries, see NATIONAL RESEARCH COUNCIL REPORT, supra note 37, at 190-93.

[27] See Des Jarlais, Chamberland, Yancovitz, Weinberg & Friedman, *Heterosexual Partners: A Large Risk Group for AIDS*, 2 LANCET 1346 (1984); Des Jarlais, Friedman, Sotheran & Stoneburner, The Sharing of drug Injection Equipment and the AIDS Epidemic in New, York City: The First Decade, in NIDA MONOCRAPH No. 80, supra note 44, at 160, 163-64; Dolan, Black, DeFord, Skinner & Rabinowitz, *Characteristics of Drug Abusers that Discrminiate Needle-Sharers*, 102 PUB. HEALTH REP. 395 (1987); Friedman, Des Jarlais & Sotheran, AIDS Health Educatioin for Intravenous Drug Users, 13 HEALTH EDUC. Q. 383, 385 (1986); Feldman & Biernacki, supra note 44, at 32-34. As one commentator put it: "Although pre-AIDS sharing of injection equipment reflected positive social relationships among IV drug users in overcoming limited supplies of injection equipment, TV drug users must now come to understand that sharing unsterilized injection equipment can lead to a protracted and painful death." Des Jarlais & Friedman, supra note 16, at 869; see Conviser & Rutledge *The Need for Innovation to Halt AIDS Among Intravenious Drug Users and Their Sexual Partners*, 3 AIDS & PUB. P6L'Y. J. 43 (1988).

[28] For economic reasons, shooting galleries are usually located in areas with a high concentration of IV drug users. Des Jarlais & Friedman, *Transmission of HIV Among Intravenous Drug Users*, in AIDS: ETIOLOGY, DIACNOSIS, TREATMENT AND PREVENTION 385 (V.T. DeVita, S. Hellman & S.A. Rosenberg eds. 1988). Also, they are more frequently located in the Northeast Corridor of the United States than on the West Coast, although San Francisco hotels where drug users gather provide a similar setting. Feldman & Biernacki, supra note 14, at 32.

[29] Des Jarlais & Friedman, supra note 57, at 385-95.

[30] Des Jarlais & Friedman, *supra* note 46, at 867; Stryker, *supra* note 40, at 722.

[31] Des Jarlais & Friedman; *supra* note 57, at 386.

[32] Des Jarlais, Friedman, Sotheran & Stoneburner, *supra* note 56, at 164; see also Hopkins, *Needle Sharing and Street Behavior* in *Response to AIDS in New York City*, in NIDA Monograph No. 80, *supra* note 44, at 18, 24 (in one study, users said they used the same needle to inject drugs 1 (19%), 2-5 (36%), 6-21 (31%), more than 21 (11%) times).

[33] The majority of shooters surveyed buys its needles from street sellers (45%) and shooting galleries (16%). Injection equipment is also obtained from doctors or pharmacies (20%) and diabetics (8%). Some sellers steal needles from hospital garbage bins or forge prescriptions, Hopkins, *supra* note 61, at 25. Some "former addicts report extensive use of 'hitters' (a person who find[s] a vessel for injection for a fee without regard for sterile technique)." D'Aquila & Williams, Epidemic Human Immunodeficiency Virus (HIV) Infection Among Intravenous Drug Users, 60 YALE J. Bio. MED. 545, 553 (1987).

[34] E.g., Des Jarlais & Friedman, *HIV Infection Among Intravenous Drug Users: Epidemiology and Risk Reduction,* 1 AIDS 67, 70 (1987); Feldman & Biernacki, supra note 14; Friedman, Des Jarlais & Sotheran, *supra* note 56, at 386 (93% of the sample knew that IV drug use was a way to get AIDS); Selwyn, Feiner, Cox, Lipshultz & Cohen, *Knowledge About AIDS and High Risk Behavior Among Intravenous Drug Abusers in New York City*, 1 AIDS 247 (1987) (97% of the

sample had accurate AIDS-related knowledge); Stimson, Donoghoe, Alldritt & Dolan, HIV Transmission Risk Behavior of clients Attending Syringe-Exchange Schemes in England and Scotland, 83 BRIT. J . ADDICTION 1449, 1451 (1988) (95% of the sample had accurate AIDS-related knowledge).

[35] Becker & Joseph, *supra* note 55. See also Ginzburg, French, Jackson, Hartsock, MacDonald & Weiss, *Health Education and Knowledge Assessment of HTLV-III Diseases Among Intravenous Drug Users*, 13 HEALTH EDUC. Q. 373, 377 (1986) (although the study shows a high level of knowledge about AIDS, the survey was unable to determine what modifications in their behavior IV drug users make based on this knowledge). Studies show that a high proportion of addicts repeatedly use the same contaminated needle, and share needles with intimate partners, dealers and casual acquaintances. Black, Dolan, DeFord, Rubinstein, Penk, Rabinowitz & Skinner, *Sharing of needles Among Users of Intravenous Drugs*, 314 NEw ENG. J. MED. 446 (1986) (those reporting sharing did so in 40% of all drug use episodes); Feldman & Biernacki, *supra* note 44, at 32 (sharing injection equipment was "common"); Hopkins, *supra* note 31 (53% of the sample report always or sometimes sharing injection equipment); Magura, Grossman, Lipton, Siddiqi, Shapiro, Marion & Amann, *Determinants of Needle Sharing Among Intravenous Drug Users*, 79 Am. J. PUB. HEALTH 459 (1989); Stimpson, Donoghoe, Aildritt & Dolan, *supra* note 63 (36% of the sample report always or sometimes sharing injection equipment); Watters, A Street-Based Outreach Model of AIDS Prevention for Intravenous Drug Users: Preliminary Evaluation, in CONTEMPORARY DRUC, PROBLEMS 411 412 (1987) (over 90% of sample said that injection equipment is typically shared). Several studies also suggest that the sexual behavior of drug users is highly resistant to change. Des Jarlais & Friedmail, *supra* note 46, at 866-67; Des Jarlais & Friedman, *supra* note 43, at 270 (five studies all found a higher percentage of intravenous drug users adopting risk-reduction activities relating to needle use than in sexual behavior).

[36] Stimson, Donoghoe, Alldritt, Dolan, *supra* note 63 (drug users in the sample reported that they shared injection equipment because of the scarcity of equipment (51%), need for a fix (50%) and/or peer influence (35%)); Becker & Joseph, *supra* note 55.

[37] Des Jarlais, Friedman & Hopkins, *Risk Reduction for the Acquired Immunodeficiency Svndrome Among Intravenous Drug Users*, 103 ANNALS INTERNAL MED. 755 (1985).

[38] D'Aquila & Williams, *supra* note 52, at 553; Des Jarlais, Friedman & Hopkins, *supra* note 66.

[39] Des Jarlais & Hopkins, Free Needles for Intravenous Drug Users at Risk for AIDS: Current Developments in New York City, 313 NEW ENG. J. MED. 23 (1985).

[40] To be sure, much of this opposition is grounded upon profound moral disapproval of the drug-dependent population and its culture. *See, e.g.*, Lambert, *Myers Opposes Needle Projects to Curb AIDS*, N.Y. Times, Apr. 10, 1990, at B4, col. 6; LaFranchi, *Texas Program on AIDS and Addicts Hits Snag*, Christian Science Monitor, Mar. 16, 1988, at 7, col. 2.

[41] Many people stereotype drug users as incapable of change. It is suggested that they do not fear, and are not concerned with I the risks of contracting HIV because they already accept significant health risks by taking drugs in the first place. In short, they are viewed as having a fatalistic acceptance of the risk of death as par-t of their lifestyle. *See, e.g.*, Beck, *Changing Behavior is a Prescription Many Still Resist*, Chicago Tribune, June 15, 1989, at 23, col. 1.
[42] Some, probably most, intravenous drug users have altered their needle-sharing behavior to avoid the risk of transmission of HIV; Des Jarlais & Friedman, *HIV and Intravenous Drug Use*, 2 AIDS S65, S65-66 (Supp. 1, 1988); Des Jarlais, Friedman & Stoneburner, *supra* note 42 at 156; Friedman, Des Jartais, Sotheran, Garber, Cohen & Smith, *AIDS and Self Organization Among Intravenous Drug Users*, 22 INT'L J. ADDICTIONs 201 (1987); Guydish, Abramowitz, Woods, Black & Sorenson, *Changes in Needle Sharing Behavior Among Intravenous Drug Users: San Francisco, 1986-1988*, 80 Am. J. PUB. HEALTH 995 (1990); Selwyn, Feiner, Cox, Lipshultz & Cohen, *Knowledge About AIDS and High Risk Behavior Among Intravenous Drug Abusers in New York City*, 1 AIDS 247 (1987). See also Centers for Disease Control, *Risk Behaviors for HIV Transmission Among Intravenous Drug Users Not in Treatment*, 39 MORB. & MORT. WKLY REP. 273 (1990); Friedman, Des Jarlais & Sotheran, *supra* note 56. Similar reductions in needle sharing are reported in Europe, including parts of Italy, France and the United Kingdom. Olievenstein, *Drug Addiction and AIDS in France in 1987*, in NIDA MONOGRAPH No. 80, *supra* note 44, at 114; Stimson, *Injecting Equipment Exchange Schemes in England and Scotland*, in NIDA MONOGRAPH No. 80, *supra* note 44, at 89; Tempesta & Di Giannantonio, *Sharing Needles and the Spread of HIV in Italy's Addict Population*, in NIDA MONOGRAPH No. 80 *supra* note 14, at 100.
[43] See *supra* note 63.
[44] *E.g.* Becker & Joseph, *supra* note 55, at 403; Des Jarlais & Friedman, *supra* note 71, at S70-1; Robertson, Skidmore & Roberts, *HIV Infection in Intravenous Drug Users: A Follow-Up Study Indicating Changes in Risk-Taking Behaviour*, 83 BRIT. J. ADDICTION 387 (1988).
[45] Des Jarlais, Friedman & Hopkins, *supra* note 65, at 758. Almost 82% of the needle sellers queried reported demand for sterile injection equipment increased since the AIDS epidemic, although only a small proportion of them attributed the increased demand directly to the AIDS epidemic.' High street prices also reflect the increased demand for sterile equipment. A 25-cent needle and syringe could cost $2.00-5.00 on the illicit market. Des Jarlais & Friedman, *supra* note 71, at S66.
[46] Des Jarlais & Friedman, *supra* note 63 at 73; Des Jarlais & Friedman, *supra* note 71, at S65 ("It is now safe to conclude that some, probably most, intravenous users will change their behavior in order to reduce their chances of developing AIDS").

Interventions to prevent HIV risk behaviors[1]

National Institute of Health Consensus statement

This Consensus Statement is not a political statement, but an independent report that resulted from research, discussions and presentations, carried out by medical and other professionals and public. In the US, as well as in many other industrialized countries, most of HIV cases account for preventable behavior, such as unsafe sex and injection practices. Thus, there is an obvious need in effective campaigns aimed at behavioral change. In preparation for the concluding observations to this statement, the effectiveness of prevention programs on HIV risk behaviors was affirmed for different populations at risk. The current debate evolves around what constitutes an effective program for a given population. It is once again asserted that there are different components to a successful HIV policy: societal, legislative, and educational. With regards to HIV prevention among drug users, professionals and public both agree that needle exchange programs, drug abuse treatment and outreach work are highly effective.

The statement concludes that it is important to get rid of legislative restrictions with regards to needle exchange programs, underlining that these barriers expose people to unnecessary risk. On the other hand, however, the Consensus Statement in its conclusion alleges the importance of drug abuse treatment as a central bulwark in the Nation's fight against AIDS.

Objective: To provide health care providers, patients, and the general public with a responsible assessment of behavioral intervention methods that may reduce the risk of HIV infection.

Participants: A non-Federal, nonadvocate, 12-member panel representing the fields of psychiatry, psychology, behavioral and social science, social work, and epidemiology. In addition, 15 experts in psychiatry, psychology, behavioral and social science, social work, and epidemiology presented data to the panel and a conference audience of 1000.

Evidence: The literature was searched through Medline and an extensive bibliography of references was provided to the panel and the conference audience. Experts prepared abstracts with relevant citations from the literature. Scientific evidence was given precedence over clinical anecdotal experience.

Consensus Process: The panel, answering predefined questions, developed its conclusions based on the scientific evidence presented in open forum and the scientific literature. The panel composed a draft statement that was read in its entirety and circulated to the experts and the audience for comment. Thereafter, the panel resolved conflicting recommendations and released a revised statement at the end of the conference. The panel finalized the revisions within a few weeks after the conference.

Conclusions: Behavioral interventions to reduce risk for HIV/AIDS are effective and should be disseminated widely. Legislative restriction on needle exchange programs must be lifted because such legislation constitutes a major barrier to realizing the potential of a powerful approach and exposes millions of people to unnecessary risk. Legislative barriers that discourage effective programs aimed at youth must be eliminated. Although sexual abstinence is a desirable objective, programs must include instruction on safer sex behaviors. The erosion of funding for drug abuse treatment programs must be halted because research data clearly show that such programs reduce risky drug abuse behavior and often eliminate drug abuse itself. Finally, new research must focus on emerging risk groups such as young people, particularly those who are gay and who are members of ethnic minority groups, and women, in whom transmission of HIV virus to their children remains a major public health problem.

INTRODUCTION

One in 250 people in the United States is infected with the human immunodeficiency virus (HIV), which causes AIDS. AIDS is the leading cause of death among men and women between the ages of 25 and 44. Every year, an additional 40,000-80,000 Americans become infected with HIV, mostly through behaviors that are preventable. In the United States, unsafe sexual behavior among men who have sex with men and unsafe injection practices among drug users still account for the largest number of cases. However, the rate of increase is greater for women than men, and there have been larger annual increases from heterosexual HIV transmission than among men who have sex with men.

The purpose of this conference was to examine what is known about behavioral interventions that are effective with different populations in different settings for the two primary modes of transmission: unsafe sexual behavior and nonsterile injection practices. Experts also provided the international and national epidemiology of HIV and a review of AIDS prevention efforts.

An extensive body of research has led to significant information on how to help individuals change their HIV-related risk behaviors. The interventions studied were based on a variety of models of behavior change, including social learning theory and related health and substance abuse models. The interventions begin with HIV and substance abuse education, but also include skill acquisition, assertiveness training, and behavioral reinforcement components. Recent research leads to the conclusion that aggressive promotion of safer sexual behavior and prevention and treatment of substance abuse could avert tens of thousands of new HIV infections and potentially save millions of dollars in health care costs. To date, however, there has not been widespread agreement among health professionals as to which interventions are most effective, in which settings, and among which populations.

Because behavioral interventions are currently the only effective way of slowing the spread of HIV infection, recommendations coming from this conference have immediate implications for service delivery in health care and educational settings, including schools; substance abuse treatment programs; community-based organizations; sexually transmitted disease clinics; inner-city health programs reaching disenfranchised high-risk women, men, and adolescents; rural health programs; and mental health programs that serve high-risk people with chronic mental illness. Knowing which behavior change interventions are most effective will assist public health personnel in allocating resources.

The conference brought together behavioral and social scientists, prevention researchers, statisticians and research methodologists, clinicians, physicians, nurses, social workers, mental health professionals, other health care professionals, and members of the public.

Following one and a half days of presentations and audience discussion, an independent, non-Federal consensus panel weighed the scientific evidence and developed a draft consensus statement that addressed following five questions:

❖ How can we identify the behaviors and contexts that place individuals/communities at risk for HIV?
❖ What individual, group, or community-based methods of intervention reduce behavioral risks? What are the benefits and risks of these procedures?
❖ Does a reduction in these behavioral risks lead to a reduction in HIV?
❖ How can risk-reduction procedures be implemented effectively?
❖ What research is most urgently needed?

How can we identify the behaviors and contexts that place individuals/communities at risk for HIV?

Major behavioral risks
Research to date has identified the key risk behaviors for HIV transmission to be unprotected anal and vaginal intercourse, having multiple sex partners, and using nonsterile drug injection equipment. Although there are some documented cases of transmission through oral-genital sexual contact, methodological issues make it difficult to precisely determine risk. At the present time, oral-genital sexual contact is considered to be a somewhat less risky behavior for contracting HIV than anal or vaginal intercourse.

Contexts that influence risk
Important social and biological contexts and cofactors increase or decrease the likelihood of risk behaviors. A major contextual influence is the prevalence of HIV itself in the local population, which greatly influences the impact of any risk behavior. Other contextual influences include: individual factors such as ace and developmental stage, early initiation of sexual behavior, sexual identity, self-esteem, untreated sexually transmitted diseases, use of alcohol, and use of other drugs, interpersonal factors such as sex with a partner of unknown HIV status, partner commitment, and negotiation of safe sex; social norms and values such as cultural and religious beliefs, gender role norms, and social inclusion versus marginalization of gay men, ethnic minorities, people of color, sex workers, women, and drug users; and political, economic, and health policy factors such as laws and regulations, employment opportunities, poverty, sexism, racism, homophobia, and availability of basic public health a tools for protective behavior, such as condoms and sterile injection equipment.

Although many of the behavioral risk factors are quite well known, the contextual risk factors are only beginning to be understood. For example, intervention programs with younger gay men need to address the fact that some of them consider HIV to be a threat mainly to older men. Negotiation about safe sex practices is much more difficult for women in populations where there are cultural barriers to doing so. Programs targeting sex workers have been highly efficacious in other countries, but in this country would encounter cultural and political barriers. The impact of poverty on seeking treatment for sexually transmitted diseases is much greater in countries without access to universal medical care. These contextual factors combine in dynamic ways to increase behavioral risk.

Means of identifying behaviors and contexts

Behavioral risks have been identified by combining data from epidemiological studies and data from studies of homosexual and heterosexual couples with only one HIV positive partner. Ongoing measurement of biomedical transmission factors will continue to be important as the, epidemic changes. Because contextual factors are more numerous and more difficult to measure than biomedical factors, a wide variety of methods have been used to identify and measure them, including qualitative, ethnographic, and observational techniques. This work is multidisciplinary and requires ongoing consultation with local community groups. Contextual information is essential for designing tailored interventions that respond to the needs and preferences of people in particular communities. In addition, if a particular intervention is not effective for some participants, this information could guide development of the next generation of interventions.

Changing trends in specific behaviors and community contexts that produce elevated risk for HIV infection

A number of established and several new and emerging behaviors and community contexts increase risk for HIV infection. In general, youth in school are showing an increase in condom use at last contact, but a trend for decreased condom use as they get older. Among gay men, the infection rate is increasing among African-American, Latino, and younger men. Injecting drug users are at increased risk because of conditions in their communities, including unavailability of sterile injecting equipment, dealer provision of infected needles, and social situations that encourage multiperson reuse of needles and other drug paraphernalia. Women, particularly women of color, recently increased dramatically as a risk group in the United States and constitute 50 percent of those infected worldwide. Much of the growth in their risk is caused by sexual contact with partners whose sexual or drug use behavior put the women at risk, vertical transmission from infected mother to infant continues to be a source of high risk for the infant, even with the treatment for mothers and infants that is now available. In addition, a variety of other special settings and subpopulations at increased risk, including incarcerated youth and adults, and individuals with chronic mental illnesses, deserve greater attention.

What individual-, group-, or community-based methods of intervention reduce behavioral risks? What are the benefits and risks of these procedures?

When we consider the entire body of literature, available knowledge converges on a clear conclusion: prevention programs have substantial effects on HIV risk behaviors. This is true across a variety of risk behaviors and in a variety of populations at risk.

Do prevention programs reduce behavioral risk?

Experts in the field have used different designs for evaluating prevention programs. The most rigorous design used in some areas of research, the randomized controlled trial, has been used in HIV prevention research but is more appropriate for testing some questions than others. For example, evaluating the effects of legislative changes would rarely be possible with randomized research. To draw its conclusions the panel examined the body of literature in a given area by considering all existing approaches to research, the strength of a given design for addressing a specific question, the number and strength of existing studies, and the convergence of effects.

Men who have sex with men

Considerable research has focused on risk reduction in men who have sex with men. Descriptive studies and nonrandomized studies with control groups show positive behavioral effects, as do randomized studies. The studies with random assignment to groups are clustered in two areas: individual interventions delivered in small group settings and programs aimed at changing community norms (e.g., using peer leaders in community settings to deliver programs). These intervention programs focus on information, skills building, self-management, problem-solving, and psychological factors such as self-efficacy and intentions. Studies with clearly defined interventions, retention of samples to allow follow-up periods as long as 18 months, and reasonable sample sizes show substantial effects for intervention over minimal intervention or control conditions. More intensive interventions (e.g., more sessions) boost efficacy.

Heterosexual transmission
Adult women at risk from sexual transmission

Data from a variety of settings demonstrate the ability to prevent HIV risk behaviors in women. A randomized trial involving a cognitive behavioral intervention aimed at inner-city women with high risk of acquiring HIV through heterosexual contact provides some of the strongest evidence of impact. Three months after intervention, women in the intervention reported a doubling of condom use from 26 percent to 56 percent for all intercourse occasions; no such change occurred for women in the comparison group. A second randomized trial, targeted at pregnant women, shows similar results at a 6-month follow-up. Results from a third randomized study yet to be published show reductions in unprotected sex and sexually transmitted diseases. A study in rural Tanzania involving treatment for sexually transmitted diseases, condom distribution, and health education found more than a 50 percent reduction in HIV seroconversion incidence over a 2-year period in women aged 15-24. Seroconversion also diminished in counseling programs for women attending a clinic in Kigali, Rwanda, and for sex workers in Bombay, India.

Couples

There is evidence that consistent and correct condom use reduces

HIV seroconversion to nearly zero in both male and female heterosexual partners. Counseling of couples in a European study was associated with large increases in protected sexual behavior.

Adolescents

The strongest support for reductions in a broad array of risky sexual behaviors comes from rigorous studies. Five randomized controlled trials used cognitive and behavioral skills training and targeted male and female, African-American, Latino, and European-American adolescents in health clinics and inner-city schools. Studies varied in sample size, and follow-ups were limited to 1 year or less, but results were consistently positive, with outcomes such as condom acquisition, condom use, and reduced number of partners.

Injection drug users

Prevention for injection drug users has involved drug abuse treatment in some cases, and outreach focused on both drug use and HIV risk behavior in others. Both approaches have been effective. Programs aimed specifically at treating drug abuse show positive effects on risk behavior and have the additional benefit of affecting drug use. These have shown minimal effects on high-risk sex. Community studies training outreach workers or using an educational media campaign to reduce the use of nonsterile needles show increased protected sexual behavior and slowing of seroconversion rates, along with impressive reductions in drug use.

Needle exchange programs

An impressive body of evidence suggests powerful effects from needle exchange programs. The number of studies showing beneficial effects on behaviors such as needle sharing greatly outnumber those showing no effects. There is no longer doubt that these programs work, yet there is a striking disjunction between what science dictates and what policy delivers. Data are available to address three central concerns:

1. Does needle exchange promote drug use? A preponderance of

evidence shows either no change or decreased drug use. The scattered cases showing increased drug use should be investigated to discover the conditions under which negative effects might occur, but these can in no way detract from the importance of needle exchange programs. Additionally, individuals in areas with needle exchange programs have increased likelihood of entering drug treatment programs.

2.Do programs encourage non-drug users, particularly youth, to use drugs? On the basis of such measures as hospitalizations for drug overdoses, there is no evidence that community norms change in favor of drug use or that more people begin using drugs. In Amsterdam and New Haven, for example, no increases in new drug users were reported after introduction of a needle exchange programs.

3.Do programs increase the number of discarded needles in the community? In the majority of studies, there was no increase in used needles discarded in public places.

There are just over 100 needle exchange programs in the United States, compared with more thin 2000 in Australia, a country with less than 10 percent of the U.S. population. Can the opposition to needle exchange programs in the United States be justified on scientific grounds? Our answer is simple and emphatic no. Studies show reduction in risk behavior is high is 80 percent in injecting drug users, with estimates of a 30 percent or greater reduction of HIV. The cost of such programs is relatively low. Needle exchange programs should be implemented at once.

Policy and large-scale interventions

As in other areas (e.g., smoking, injury control), policy interventions can remove barriers to protective behavior. In the United States and other countries, such interventions have resulted in dramatic reductions in risk behavior. In Connecticut, for example, a single legislative action legalizing over-the-counter purchase of sterile injection equipment led to an immediate and profound reduction in the sharing of nonsterile needles. A national campaign in Switzerland to promote the use of condoms dramatically reduced risky sexual behavior. Regulations on the use of condoms by sex workers in Thailand also led to fewer unprotected sex acts. The results thus far have been impressive. Given the potential benefit of policy changes, these should be implemented as local circumstances allow and, once implemented, should be evaluated as often and thoroughly as possible

Issues in need of further work
Populations and settings
A promising start has been made to reduce risk in persons often marginalized. Homeless, chronically mentally ill, runaway, incarcerated, HIV-positive, and physically and developmentally challenged persons face obstacles that affect their ability to initiate and maintain behavior change. In addition, little is known about the risk behaviors of lesbians and bisexual women, heterosexual men, persons over 50 years old, and sexually active youth.

African-American and Latino communities experience disproportionate infection. The application of culturally appropriate strategies demands ethnographic research to understand values, attitudes, behaviors, and factors such as socioeconomic status in different communities. Cultural factors may affect the ability of individuals to change behavior. Researchers from different ethnic or cultural backgrounds may help address this issue. Language and cultural barriers to delivery of interventions must be addressed, with special consideration for individuals whose physical or other impairments limit access to most programs.

Prenatal care and sexually transmitted disease clinics are proven to be effective settings for delivery of HIV intervention. Further research is needed in these and other medical settings. In addition, individuals in institutions such as prisons and mental health facilities, and those in remote areas, require special attention.

Maintenance, generalizability, and theory

Understanding and evaluating the maintenance of behavior change requires multivariate, longitudinal studies. In this way, changes in patterns of behavior and causal associations can be estimated. Long-term follow-up of subjects is necessary. Similarly, more attention to generalizability is needed. An intervention proven effective in one city may not be applicable in another city with a similar population but with different community norms. Methodological issues in need of additional attention include research strategies that measure and enhance validity of self-report, standardization of risk behavior questions and questioning techniques, comparability of intervention conditions across different studies, examining participants and nonresponders to an intervention, and measuring changes in multiple risk profiles over time.

A developmental framework may be helpful for considering the origins of HIV risk behavior. Efforts are needed to incorporate knowledge of childhood antecedents of HIV risk behaviors in adolescents. Can early intervention that alters these antecedents reduce or delay HIV risk behaviors? The body of research now being done to reduce already existing risk behaviors such as unprotected sex and drug use needs to be linked with other research traditions that target antecedents of HIV risk behaviors.

Impact and cost-effectiveness

Reviews on HIV prevention conclude that programs produce significant effects, but a statistical advantage may not necessarily equate to meaningful change. An example comes from a study on condom use in more than 13,000 injecting drug users. An intervention nearly doubled consistent condom use, from a baseline level of 10 percent to 19 percent. Although the change was significant from a public health perspective, 81 percent of this high-risk population still engaged in high-risk sexual behavior. This highlights the importance of examining and improving impact as well as assessing statistical significance. Impact is assessed by understanding the efficacy of an intervention, the magnitude of behavior change, and the influence of this change on seroconversion.

A key issue is the degree to which the field has confronted the issue of efficacy (impact of interventions in controlled circumstances) versus effectiveness (effects in real-world setting). Little effectiveness research has been done. This limits the ability to estimate the impact likely to occur if the current generation of risk-reduction strategies, proven useful in efficacy trials, were applied on a large scale outside the research setting. The panel concluded that HIV prevention research is mature enough that some, but not all interventions, are ready for tests of effectiveness. This will require different research strategies and the involvement of professionals from additional disciplines beyond those used for efficacy trials.

The cost-effectiveness of interventions is an important issue in decisions about resource allocation. Research thus far has been positive, but more research is needed to examine the costs and benefits of HIV risk prevention programs.

Behavioral issues arising from biomedical advances
Important advances in medicine have created new and pressing behavioral issues. Pharmacologic treatment of HIV-positive individuals may increase longevity, but it is not known how such successfully treated individuals will alter their recreational drug use or sexual behavior. Complicated medical regimens raise issues of adherence, with the possibility that incomplete adherence will lead to resistant strains of the virus. Studies of biochemical preventive treatment after sexual exposure to HIV raise questions about risk-reduction counseling. For example, will individuals feel free to engage in risky sex as post-exposure treatment becomes more an option?

Pharmacologic treatment profiles now exist to reduce transmission of HIV from mother to newborn child. This demonstrated preventive intervention offers new opportunities to study behavioral issues and barriers to access in a new and important context.

Policy

Current evidence suggests that some of the most powerful positive effects on HIV risk behavior have been produced by legislative and regulatory changes. One need look no further than to the experience in Connecticut, where one legislative action permitting the purchase of sterile injection equipment had an immediate and pronounced effect on behavior. Here we see the potentially low cost and high effectiveness of intervention at the policy level. Policymaking can be conceptualized as behavior, and as such can and should be studied. Social policy, legal change, and community mobilization are powerful means of intervention and must be a legitimate area of inquiry at the National Institutes of Health and the Centers for Disease Control and Prevention.

Several examples beyond the Connecticut experience show the power of policy changes. Australia, for instance, has a low rate of HIV despite population profiles in some areas similar to profiles in areas in the United States that have high HIV seroconversion rates. Cities such as Tacoma, Toronto, Sydney, Glasgow, and Lund have kept the HIV infection rate low, coincident with policies making sterile needles available for injecting drug users, boosting education aimed at risk reduction, making condoms more available, and enhancing programs for the treatment of sexually transmitted diseases. Impressive results have been reported from around the world on government action to reduce risk and infection in many populations at risk.

Little qualitative and quantitative research has been done in HIV prevention policy, and no body of evidence exists to inform the field about the factors that influence policy, where policy intervention is most likely to be effective, and how best to encourage policy and legislative changes. We believe that funding should be devoted to the study of policy and legislative changes and that national, state, and local levels be considered.

Of utmost importance is that HIV prevention policy be based, whenever possible, on scientific information. This occurs too little - the behavior placing the public health at greatest risk may be occurring in legislative and other decision-making bodies. The Federal ban on funding for needle exchange programs as well as restrictions on selling injection equipment are absolutely contraindicated and erect formidable barriers to implementing what is known to be effective. Many thousands of unnecessary deaths will occur as a result.

The single greatest increase in HIV prevention funding occurred with 1996 Federal legislation in the United States providing $50 million within block grant entitlements for programs teaching adolescents abstinence from sexual behavior. Among the criteria for programs funded through the block grant program are the following two requirements: (1) "has as its exclusive purpose, teaching the social psychological, and health gains to be realized by abstaining from sexual activity" and (2) "teaches that a mutually faithful monogamous relationship in the context of marriage is the expected standard of human sexual activity" (Public Health Service Act, Public Law 104-193, Sec. 912). Some programs based on an abstinence model propose that approaches such as the use of condoms are ineffective. This model places policy in direct conflict with science because it ignores overwhelming evidence that other programs are effective. Abstinence-only programs cannot be justified in the face of effective programs and given the fact that we face an international emergency in the AIDS epidemic.

Another instance of policy conflicting with knowledge is in providing treatment for drug abuse. Research shows that treatment of drug abusers with methadone maintenance, outpatient drug-free treatments, residential treatment, or detoxification not only decreases drug use but has a substantial effect on risk behaviors (use of shared needles and protected sex). At the same time that this knowledge has reached a critical mass, funding of drug treatment programs has been reduced in many localities. This tragic trend must be reversed.

Policy and legislative change can have rapid, powerful, and positive results. This key area of the field has been given little attention, a problem that needs remedy. A coordinated effort is needed, and the Government must take strong and immediate steps to protect its citizens. Drawing together legal and policy changes and program implementation occurring at international, national, and local levels offers great promise. Strong political leadership is necessary to direct this effort. The United States has much to learn from other countries where political leaders have taken this issue seriously and, by supporting vigorous prevention strategies, have prevented even more tragedy from occurring from AIDS.

Does a reduction in these behavioral risks lead to a reduction in HIV?

The evidence is unequivocal that consistent and effective use of condoms and of sterile injecting equipment on the part of injection drug users is nearly 100 percent effective in protecting against HIV. Reduction in risky behavior leads to reduction in HIV to a degree that depends on context, particularly the local prevalence of HIV infection.

It is important to keep HIV seroincidence in mind as the ultimate outcome of interest for HIV prevention efforts. Seroincidence estimates also allow us to compare effectiveness and cost of different programs. Direct measurement of HIV infection is a feasible and desirable outcome variable for some programs. However, practical, ethical, and fiscal barriers often make reliance on measured seroconversion undesirable. In these instances, proxy indices - including other biological markers or modeled estimates of seroincidence based on behavioral outcomes - can be used to estimate the effects of prevention programs on seroincidence.

Study designs that lend themselves to using seroconversions as an outcome

To find reliable differences between intervention and control or comparison samples, one must expect a minimum number of seroconversions in the control sample within the time frame of the study. These are found in populations where seroconversion rates are high, in large samples, or in studies with long followup. Only a limited number of situations have lent themselves to clinical trials and other studies on this scale.

Many studies using seroincidence as a measure of outcome were conducted in developing countries where HIV incidence is high and policy interventions or community-level programs have been implemented. Among these are studies from Tanzania and Bombay with comparison populations and from Thailand, where an historical comparison was employed. Few studies in the United States have used HIV or any biological measure as an endpoint for the reasons cited above. In the United States and elsewhere, seroconversion has been used to measure the effect of sterile injection equipment availability, bleach cleaning interventions, and methadone treatment with injecting drug users.

Constraints on using seroconversion outcomes

Although seroconversion is a preferred standard for intervention efficacy, there are practical and ethical obstacles to its use. For example, there is a potential selective dropout of research participants who will not agree to repeated HIV testing, Furthermore, research costs can be greatly increased by pre- and post-test counseling and followup or referral for research subjects who are identified as HIV-positive in the study. Counseling and referral are, of course, required by ethical research practice. Nevertheless, where possible and feasible, it is important that behavioral and policy interventions be validated using seroincidence as an outcome.

Transmission models to estimate effects of behavioral outcomes on HIV infection rates

When HIV seroconversion outcomes are not feasible, well-designed self-report behavioral outcomes have shown indications of being valid and reliable. These behavioral outcomes can be employed in transmission models to estimate the number of averted cases. The models have been developed from studies of HIV-discordant couples and epidemiological studies. Although use of these models requires assumptions about future prevalence and about relationships among variables being studied, a reasonable range of estimates about the probable impact of the intervention on HIV can thus be generated. In theory, estimates of HIV seroconversion during the study may be extended into the future under varying estimates of the maintenance of positive behavioral outcome. The models may also be extended to estimate the potential impact were the program more widely implemented in similar contexts. Finally, potential effects on seroconversion in field settings may be estimated, using these models, from data on behavioral outcomes from studies done in research settings. These models can estimate the impact on seroconversion using reasonable assumptions that the interventions will have less effectiveness in field settings.

Estimates of the effects of behavioral outcomes on HIV seroconversion are still relatively few and mostly retrospective. It should be possible to produce such estimates in advance of prevention trials, continent on the targeted magnitude of behavioral outcomes and the expected prevalence of HIV infection in the local population. We recommend that such estimates be employed as an additional outcome measure for trials with behavioral endpoints whenever possible. Ongoing, work on these models is needed to update and improve the database used to produce and validate them. Furthermore, there is a need to validate, by use of empirical data, the assumption that transmission rates based on naturally occurring behaviors are equivalent to transmission rates based on behavioral changes in response to prevention efforts. These models can also be used to estimate the validity of self-reports.

Other biological markers as surrogates for HIV seroconversion
Incidence of certain sexually transmitted diseases has been used as a plausible surrogate for HIV seroconversion. The same sexual behaviors are risks for HIV and some sexually transmitted diseases. Sexually transmitted diseases are a powerful potentiator of HIV sereconversion in exposed persons. The higher incidence of sexually transmitted diseases also makes detection of program effects more sensitive. Two ongoing multicenter randomized controlled

trials for heterosexual populations have chosen incidence of sexually transmitted diseases as a biologic marker to study the efficacy of HIV prevention interventions, as have international studies such as the study in Tanzania. Unpublished results of a Centers for Disease Control and Prevention project show a decrease in the rate of sexually transmitted diseases to be correlated with a decrease in HIV-related risk behavior. Hepatitis C has been used effectively as a biological marker in studies involving injecting drug user populations, because of overlapping transmission routes. Sexually transmitted disease incidence, hepatitis C incidence, and other infectious disease incidence are reasonable markers for expected HIV exposure.

How can risk-reduction procedures be implemented effectively?

Studies ready for implementation

A number of interventions have been evaluated in current research and are ready to be implemented within communities. Indeed, some are already being implemented by health departments and community-based organizations. Interventions at the individual level include the following:

❖ Outreach, needle exchange activities, treatment programs, and face-to-face counseling programs for substance-abusing populations

❖ Cognitive-behavioral small group, face-to-face counseling, and skills-building (proper condom use, negotiation, refusal) programs for men who have sex with men

❖ Cognitive-behavioral small group, face-to-face counseling, and skills building (i.e., proper condom use, negotiation, refusal) programs for women that pay special attention to their concerns (e.g., child care, transportation, and relationships with significant others)

❖ Condom distribution and testing and treatment for sexually transmitted diseases for sex workers and other sexually active individuals at high risk for sexually transmitted diseases

❖ Cognitive-behavioral educational and skills-building groups for youth and adolescents in various settings.

At the family or dyad level, interventions include counseling for couples (including HIV-serodiscordant couples) in both the United States and other countries. Within the community, interventions include changing community norms through community outreach and opinion leaders for men who have sex with men as well as injection drug-using networks.

At the policy level there are a number of strategies:

❖ Lifting government restrictions on needle exchange programs
❖ Providing increased government funding for drug and alcohol treatment programs, including methadone maintenance
❖ Support for sex education interventions that focus beyond abstinence
❖ Lifting constraints on condom availability (e.g., in correctional facilities).

Implementation considerations

Several factors may influence implementation of HIV risk behavior interventions within the United States.

First, compliance with interventions is improved when targeted individuals are involved at every phase of the process of conceptualization, development, and implementation of the programs. Input of these individuals is needed to help solve this health crisis.

Second, programs need to be cultural sensitive. This requires attention not only to ethnicity and language but also to other factors including social class, age, developmental stage, and sexual orientation.

Third, an appropriate intervention dosage must be selected for the population; this includes the number, length, and intensity of the intervention. Studies demonstrate that numerous intervention points over extended periods of time are more efficacious than once-only approaches for most populations. Almost all reported studies have short follow-up (3-18 months), which suggests that attention must be paid to maintenance efforts. It may be necessary to include additional, periodic intervention points for subsets of the population; longer-term follow-up would assist in determining this fact.

Fourth, when HIV risk behavior interventions are being introduced, it is important to address community myths. For example, scientifically derived results do not support assertions that needle exchange programs will lead to increased needle-injecting behavior among current users or an increase in the number of users. Nor do the data indicate that sex education programs result in earlier onset of sexual behavior or more sexual partners, or that condom distribution fosters more risky behavior. To the contrary, outcomes of these programs are quite consistent with the values of most communities. For example, behavioral interventions lead injecting drug users to inject less frequently, and the number of users in a community may decrease; after interventions, young people tend to delay initiation of intercourse or, if they are sexually active, have fewer partners; and adults, following intervention, engage in fewer incidents of risky sexual behavior. Armed with this knowledge, those who implement programs should confidently solicit the support and involvement of local government, educational, and religious leaders.

Despite notable gains relevant to implementation of prevention programs, very little cost analysis information has been available to guide community-based organizations, State and local health departments, and other practitioners. These analyses are important in determining the most cost-effective interventions for implementation. In addition, communities lack fiscal resources to support such interventions once they are proven successful. Finally, there are social and cultural barriers to implementation of programs; these include homophobia, gender inequality, and racism.

Sufficient training of personnel, monitoring of procedures to ensure fidelity to key components and established methods, and strong evaluation plans are essential components of any implementation strategy. When training and local capacity-building are necessary for implementation, training and technical assistance should be available to facilitate prevention programs at state and local levels. Evaluation results should be reported and widely disseminated so as to advance both science and practice. Newly implemented programs yielding results different from established findings should be carefully compared with original designs in order to explain the variance in outcomes.

The next step

Just as the Food and Drug Administration conditionally approves experimental drugs in emergency situations, so should policymakers support active dissemination of the most promising programs at this time based on the urgency of the AIDS epidemic. A critical issue that must be addressed involves the criteria for choosing interventions most ready for implementation in the community. The most obvious is evidence of strong program effects observed under rigorous, controlled research conditions. Among programs with strong effects, priority should be given to interventions that can be delivered with high reliability and fidelity to the original program model. Usually such programs do not require significant new demands or elaborate training at the delivery site.

At this next stage there will nevertheless be programs that show promise but still require additional research to ensure their effectiveness. At least two criteria should be considered in choosing promising programs for further evaluation. First, programs that show strong short-term effects but lack long-term results should be studied to estimate their long-term effectiveness. Second, programs that have shown promising effects for only a very narrowly defined range of settings or conditions of implementation should be studied to assess the generalizability of their effectiveness in other settings and contexts.

Numerous other interventions developed solely by community organizations were not described during the consensus development conference by the researchers, yet were brought to the attention of the panel by the public statements at the conference by community activists and practitioners. The efficacy of these approaches has not been demonstrated through careful evaluation. However, because community workers have developed a number of innovative and promising programs, there is a great need for them to work together with researchers to further HIV risk behavior intervention science and practice.

What research is most urgently needed

The most urgently needed research is that which is essential for containing the HIV/AIDS epidemic. In particular, we need to track emerging behavioral risk factors and to aim preventive procedures at these risk factors with as much precision as possible.

Tracking emerging risk

A most urgent area for research is in developing improved methods of identifying emerging risks within large populations. For example, in the United States we need to know as early as possible what settings, regions, and subpopulations are likely to show increases in seroconversion to HIV The best strategy for this identification is to track increases in known behavioral risks, which when combined with sufficiently high HIV prevalence predicts regions of particular vulnerability. Regional strategies are needed for regularly tracking increases in these behaviors in order to effectively offer known prevention strategies before seroconversion occurs. These regional strategies must be coordinated with the National HIV tracking system. Research is needed on how to collect this information regionally. How can studies collect representative data/behavioral information from regional populations in ways that are fully acceptable to the local communities involved? This regional strategy of risk tracking can draw on two areas of established research. First, clearly established risky behaviors serve as reliable harbingers of seroconversion. These include behaviors that directly increase the likelihood of HIV transmission, such as unprotected sex and needle sharing and practices that make these behaviors more likely, such as alcohol abuse in adolescents. Second, methods for inquiring about these risky behaviors have been established and validated. Careful evaluation of the most cost-efficient approaches to regional tracking is needed, as well as approaches to ensure that strategies used are compatible with community values and maximum effectiveness.

Young people

The epidemic in the United States is currently shifting to young people, particularly those who are gay, members of racial and ethnic minorities, and out-of-school adolescents. Because adolescents may be at risk for HIV infection in their early to mid teens, it is important to establish interventions for youth at an earlier age before the onset of risk behavior (sexual activity and drug use). Thus, the U.S. program of research must give highest priority to providing effective prevention programs for these subpopulations. Programs already shown to be effective for these subpopulations must be improved to ensure long-term maintenance of the reduction in risky behavior. Current interventions should be widely disseminated, and improved interventions, as they become available, should quickly replace those that have been less effective. Dissemination should include careful training of providers, monitoring to ensure fidelity of delivery, continuous evaluation of effectiveness, and modification where required by community and cultural needs and circumstances.

HIV-positive individuals

Effective interventions with people who are HIV positive can enable them to practice safer sex and safer needle use and thus help to contain the HIV epidemic. There is a startling paucity of well-developed interventions specifically designed for HIV-positive persons. Moreover, as biological treatment for those who are HIV positive improves, the need for these preventive services will become even more pressing.

Women

It is essential to continue development of interventions to reduce heterosexual transmission of HIV to women as well as their risk of drug abuse behavior. These interventions should focus on the effect of community expectations of women and power differentials in their relationships with men. Moreover, additional research with female condoms and microbicides may facilitate preventive interventions that enhance women's control of exposure to HIV risk.

Linking scientific findings to law and policy
Most urgent is the need to rapidly bridge the serious gap that is widening between clear scientific results and the law and policies of the United States, As this statement has noted forcefully, there is clear scientific evidence supporting needle exchange programs, drug abuse treatment, and interventions with adolescents as essential components of our National program to contain the AIDS epidemic. Even as evidence rapidly accumulates on the success of these programs, however, legislation has been passed to make provision of these interventions extremely difficult. There is no more urgent need than to remedy this dangerous chasm. National leaders, legislators, scientists, and service providers must unite to understand fully this growing catastrophe. Why are voters unaware of these issues? What pressures and circumstances of government make it unresponsive to these compelling public health needs and effective programs? What are the limits in scientific communication that may obscure the legislative import of these scientific findings?

Conclusions and recommendations
1. Preventive interventions are effective for reducing behavioral risk for HIV/AIDS and must be widely disseminated. Their application in practice settings may require careful training of personnel, close monitoring of the fidelity of procedures, and on-going monitoring of effectiveness. Results of this evaluation must be reported; and where effectiveness in field settings is reduced, program modifications must be undertaken immediately. Three approaches are particularly effective for risk in drug abuse behavior: needle exchange programs, drug abuse treatment, and outreach programs

for drug abusers not enrolled in treatment. Several programs were deemed effective for risky sexual behavior. These programs include (1) information about HIV/AIDS and (2) building skills to use condoms and to negotiate the interpersonal challenges of safer sex. Effective safer sex programs have been developed for men who have sex with men, for women, and for adolescents.

2. The epidemic in the United States is shifting to young people, particularly those who are gay and who are members of ethnic minority groups. New research must focus on these emerging risk groups. Interventions must be developed and perfected, and special attention must be given to long-term maintenance of effects. In addition, AIDS is steadily increasing in women, and transmission of HIV virus to their children remains a major public health problem. Interventions focused on their special needs are essential.

3. Regional tracking of changes in behavioral risk will be necessary to identify settings, subpopulations, and geographical regions with special risk for seroconversion to HIV-positive status as the epidemic continues to change. This effort, if properly coordinated with national tracking strategies, could play a critical part in a U.S. strategy to contain the spread of HIV.

4. Programs must be developed to help individuals already infected with HIV to avoid risky sexual and substance abuse behavior. This National priority will become more pressing as new biological treatments prolong life. Thus, prevention programs for HIV-positive people must have outcomes that can be maintained over long periods of time, in order to slow the spread of infection.

5. Legislative restriction on needle exchange programs must be lifted. Such legislation constitutes a major barrier to realizing the potential of a powerful approach and exposes millions of people to unnecessary risk.

6. Legislative barriers that discourage effective programs aimed at youth must be eliminated. Although sexual abstinence is a desirable objective, programs must include instruction in safe sex behavior, including condom use. The effectiveness of these programs is supported by strong scientific evidence. However, they are discour-

aged by welfare reform provisions, which support only programs using abstinence as the only goal.

7. The erosion of funding for drug and alcohol abuse treatment programs must be halted. Research data are clear that the programs reduce risky drug and alcohol abuse behavior and often eliminate drug abuse itself. Drug and alcohol abuse treatment is a central bulwark in the nation's defense against HIV/AIDS.

8. The catastrophic breach between HIV/AIDS prevention science and the legislative process must be healed. Citizens, legislators, political leaders, service providers, and scientists must unite so that scientific data may properly inform legislative process. The study of policy development, the impact of policy, and policy change must be supported by federal agencies.

NOTES

[1] This statement was originally published as: Interventions to Prevent HIV Risk Behaviors. 1997 February 11-13;15(2): 1-41.

For making bibliographic reference to consensus statement no. 104 in the electronic forr-n displayed here, it is recommended that the following format be used: Interventions to Prevent HIV Risk Behaviors. NIH Consensus Statement Online 1997 Feb 11-13; 15(2): 1-41.

NIH Consensus Statements are prepared by a nonadvocate, non-Federal panel of experts, based on (1) presentations by investigators working in areas relevant to the consensus questions during a 2-day public session; (2) questions and statements from conference attendees during open discussion periods that are part of the public session; and (3) closed deliberations by the panel during the remainder of the second day and morning of the third. This statement is an independent report of the consensus panel and is not a policy statement of the NIH or the Federal Government.

CONSENSUS DEVELOPMENT PANEL

David Reiss, M.D.
Panel and Conference Chairperson
Professor and Director
Division of Research
Department of Psychiatry and Behavioral Science
George Washington University Medical Center
Washington, DC

C. Hendricks Brown, Ph.D.
Professor
Department of Epidemiology and Biostatistics
College of Public Health
University of South Florida
Tampa, Florida

Kelly D. Brownell, Ph.D.
Professor of Psychology, Epidemiology, and Public Health
Director of the Yale Center for Eating and Weight Disorders
Master of Silliman College
Yale University
Department of Psychology
New Haven, Connecticut

Patricia Cohen, Ph.D.
Professor
Division of Epidemiology
Department of Psychiatry
Columbia University
New York, New York

Julia R. Heiman, Ph.D.
Professor
Department of Psychiatry and Behavioral Sciences
University of Washington
Outpatient Psychiatry Center
Seattle, Washington

Richard H. Price, Ph.D.
Professor of Psychology and Research Scientist
Department of Psychology
Institute for Social Research
University of Michigan
Ann Arbor, Michigan

Sohail Rana, M.D.
Associate Professor
Director, Pediatric HIV Service
Department of Pediatrics
Howard University Hospital
Washington, DC

Edward Seidman, Ph.D.
Professor
Department of Psychology
Center for Community Research and Action
New York University
New York, New York

Mickey W Smith, B.A.S.W
Manager, Scott-Harper Recovery House
Mental Health and Addictions Treatment
Services
Whitman-Walker Clinic, Inc.
Washington, DC

HIV/AIDS and the Drug Culture: Shattered Lives[1]

by Elizabeth Hagan RN, Patient Care Coordinator,
Hospice Care of Rhode Island & Joan Gormley RN,
Immunology Center, the Miriam Hospital, Providence, RI

There are different models to address illicit drug use, ranging from those aiming at the total elimination of the problem, to those embracing the pragmatic prevention approaches. The "crime and punishment" model implies incarcerating (or punishing) those who engage in legally unacceptable behaviors, however, the life itself shows that this model doesn't seem to work. The restriction model is discarded due to its inability to secure trust between those who preach it and those are being preached, as it consists of mixed messages that often contradict each other. The "all or nothing" approach to drug use may seem simple and logical, but it includes detoxification and an extensive inpatient program, producing more failures than successes The harm reduction model can be an effective alternative to the above-mentioned approaches. Its principles are based on compassion and understanding, on the fact that drugs are here to stay and the problem cannot be eliminated and thus it requires non-biased and non-judgemental approach.

"THE SCOPE OF THE ISSUE"

At one time the interaction between injecting drug users and the health care system was limited to acute medical issues, such as cellulitis, pneumonia, endocarditis, and drug overdose. Health care providers gave little thought to an individual's chronic medical problems. The HIV epidemic dramatically changed this situation (Wartenberg and Samet, 1992).

One of the largest causes of HIV transmission in the United States is the sharing of needles and syringes for the injection of drugs. It has led to over 205,000 documented cases of AIDS. At least twice as many whites as African-Americans inject drugs, but injection-related HIV transmission disproportionately affects communities of color. African-American and Latino communities face a public health crisis. If we combine data on AIDS and drug use, we find that among those who inject drugs, African Americans are four times as likely as whites to get AIDS (Day, 1997). In 1996 almost 100,000 African Americans had injecton-related AIDS or had died from AIDS. AIDS is the leading cause of death among twenty-four to forty-four-year-old Latinos in the United States; more than half of those deaths are injection-related. The AIDS death rate for Latinos in this age group is more than double that of whites in the same age group (Day, 1997). Latinos are three times more likely to contract AIDS than to die from an overdose.

Several models are currently being used to address illicit drug use, which, according to statistics, have not been successful.

THE MIXED MESSAGE MODEL

When the use of alcohol, tobacco, and prescription, over-the-counter, and illicit drugs are included, almost no one in our society is truly drug-free (Duncan et al., 1994). The "just say no to drugs" model, which declares all drugs bad, has failed to make clear that drugs are neither good nor bad and contradicts the current pervasive drug use in society. Elementary-school age children are confused by this mixed message when they observe treatment for them-selves or others with multiple medications. In an effort to discour-age illegal drug use, risks and dangers are often exaggerated. Young adults are distrustful because the message is not truthful and causes suspicion regarding information about addiction. Marijuana may not have made them seek out cocaine or heroin. The typical response of adolescents and young adults to such contradictory information is simply to discredit the message.

THE CRIME AND PUNISHMENT MODEL

The United States spends 65 percent of its drug intervention dol-lars on incarceration and prosecution, and a mere 35 percent on education, prevention, research and treatment combined. Theoretically this means if the criminal model was successful, drug use would be reduced by 65 percent. In fact, drug use has steadily increased according to the most current household survey by the National Institute of Drug Abuse (Department of Health and Human Services, 1997).

"FATHER KNOWS BEST" MODEL

This disease model prescribes that tile intravenous drug user (IDU) must first be detoxified and then taught healthier coping mecha-nisms. Detoxification can be done either in an inpatient or outpa-tient program. The length of an inpatient program varies from as little as three days to as long as two months and the availability of beds is limited. An outpatient program can last as long as a year. Approximately 10 percent of tile drug-using population enter detoxification programs. The remaining 90 percent includes those who cannot participate because of lack of space and those who do not wish to enter these facilities. Recovery from drug use is not a constant progression. Rather, it involves occasionally falling back a few steps before moving forward again. This model is an all-or-nothing approach that produces more failures than successes.

A new model that has gained interest recently is based on the principle of reducing the risks to both tile patient and the community.

THE HARM REDUCTION MODEL

Harm reduction is a model of care that emerged from the need for an alternative treatment for injection drug users. The theory focuses on maximizing community health interventions that promote safety and reduce drug-related harm. It is a community-based, public health intervention model that provides support and health promotion services to drug users without the requirement that the requirement that they remain drug-free (Duncan, 1995). This is a radical change from the abstinence-oriented perspective, It requires that one must first accept the individual's choice to use drugs. In using this model of care, the health care professional acknowledges the client's responsibility for his or her own choices. The harm reduction model is based on the following principles:

❖ All humans have intrinsic value and dignity.
❖ All have the right to comprehensive nonjudgemental medical and social services.
❖ Licit and illicit drugs are neither good nor bad.
❖ Users are competent to make choices.
❖ Outcomes are in the hands of the patient.
❖ Options are provided in a nonjudgmental, noncoercive way.

Intrinsic value and dignity are the basis of the professional health care model that is nondiscriminating regardless of the disease. One does not judge a patient with HIV any more or less than one would judge a person with cardiac disease or cancer,

Acknowledging a person's value and dignity is the basis of a trusting relationship that is equally rewarding to both parties. It is the foundation for building the strongest possible positive relationship with a client.

Nonjudgmental medical and social services for comprehensive care of an individual create an atmosphere of caring and concern for the person's well-being. It addresses the whole patient rather than the drug use issue. Drugs have alwavs been and are likely to remain a part of American Culture. Drug use will happen. Instead of becoming morally indignant and punitive, we call assume the existence of drug use and seek to minimize its negative effects (Rosenbaum, 1997).

Users are competent to make choices. Just as any other patient or client, a person who uses drugs is capable of making choices, participating in his or her health care and selecting the best plan of care with the chosen health care provider. Abstinence should never be a criterion for receiving care. The client's and health care professional's goal should be to create a partnership based on appropriate behavior, not sobriety (Lyons, 1996). Outcomes are in the hands of the patient. Assessing and addressing tile patients' needs with information, referrals, and options acknowledges their right to determine what results they would like to achieve and what method they would like to employ to gain the results. The responsibility is with the individual.

Although providing options in a nonjudgmental, noncoercive way is a familiar concept in the health care field, it call be difficult to put into practice. Some words set tip a hostile, adversarial environment. The terms "noncompliant," "drug seeking," and "difficult" reflect personal judgment by a nurse or social worker. Better terms for describing behaviors would be nonadherent or "challenging." The providers' feelings about drug use need to be set aside. The user has a wealth of information that a nonuser needs to learn. The greatest educator on drug use is the patient. Information about illicit drug use, routes of administration, types of drugs used, availability, cost, and methods of payment are a necessary part of the assessment plan. The question, "What can you tell me about heroin use in this area?" will reveal important opportunities for interventions. The plan of care will vary if the drug of choice is heroin, crack, cocaine, or amphetamines. The answers to these questions provide health care professionals with information to suggest ways the client will be able to reduce harm while promoting safety and wellness.

Legal syringe exchange and accessible sterile drug-using and safer-sex equipment are the top priorities in reducing tile transmission of the HIV virus. The effectiveness of this barren reduction approach is evident when the statistics from Australia are reviewed. There a needle exchange program has been in place for ten years, and the result his been a reduction in the seroprevalence of HIV among drug users from 50 percent to 2 percent.

Needles and syringes are not designed for reuse. They are difficult to completely clean and disinfect. The only reliable ways to prevent transmission of HIV are to either stop injecting drugs or stop sharing equipment. Needle exchange programs hold promise as an effective intervention to limit HIV transmission,

Despite the fact that access to sterile needles through needle exchange programs has been shown to reduce the transmission of HIV/AIDS among IDUs and their families, there is currently a ban on federal funding for such programs. Only 117 needle exchange programs currently operate in approximately seventy-two cities, relying mainly on volunteers. The ban exists despite seven federally sponsored reports attesting to the efficacy of clean needle exchange for reducing HIV transmission among drug users. Study after study has shown that needle exchange does not lead to an increase in illegal drug use, nor does it lead to new drug users, As an example, a study in Connecticut found that new HIV infections were reduced by 33 percent among needle exchange participants over a yearlong period.

Needle exchange programs provide a critical link between IDUs and public health services because workers often refer addicts to treatment programs. A recent study estimated conservatively that from 1987 to 1995 up to 10,000 HIV infections could have been prevented by a national program of needle exchange (Lurie and Drucker, 1997). The cost to the U.S. health care system of treating these preventable cases is an estimated $500 million. The average

cost of operating a needle exchange program that can provide services to hundreds is $169,000 a year. The final irony is the com-
parison between this figure and the average lifetime cost of treating
one person infected with HIV/AIDS, $119,000.

In 1997 an independent consensus panel convened by National
Institutes of Health found that "an impressive body of evidence
suggests powerful effects from needle-exchange programs ... there
is no longer doubt that these programs work." Yet, despite this epidemic, tile United States remains one of the few industrialised
countries that refuses to provide easy access to sterile syringes
(Editorial, 1998).

HIV/AIDS is a public health problem without a contemporary
parallel. As health care providers become more informed about
transmission by intravenous drug use, more and more each year are
becoming involved in the prevention and reduction of harm to
individuals, families, and communities by volunteering, speaking,
and engaging in political actions supporting needle exchange in
the United States.

NOTES

[1] Originally printed in E. Hagan and J. Gormley *HIV/AIDS and the Drug
Culture: Shattered Lives* (Binghamton, NY: The Haworth Press, Inc) 1998
pp 3-8. Used with permission.

Part 2
Policy Aspects

*We have divided the debate section of this book into
two broad areas, policy aspects and human rights aspects.
The policy aspects deal with particularly pragmatic concerns
such as "Are we winning the war against drugs?" or even
"Is the war against drugs winnable?" Other aspects might
include "Does drug prohibition work or should we focus
on another way to decrease drug use?" Of course, the
background readings might help clarify some of these
issues for you. At the end of each reading there are
debate/discussion questions that can act as starting
points for further reflection and discussion.*

The Control of Drugs[1]

by Michael Gossop, Head of Research,
Drug Dependency Unit, Maudsley Hospital, London.

Many philosophers and legal scholars have dedicated their works to the limit of state control over one's liberty and discussion of whether there should be any limitations to personal freedom. John Stuart Mill in his work "On Liberty" that was published in 1859 strongly argued in favor of individual autonomy and the limited power of the state, and came to the following conclusion: Over himself, over his own body and mind, the individual is sovereign.

Mill's theory when applied to the prohibitionist policies whether it is with regards to alcohol or drugs, demonstrates how policies, that are only morally motivated and that lack reasoned arguments and scientific evidence fail their primary goals to prevent members of a community from engaging in the "wrong" behavior. During the thirteen years of American alcohol prohibition, more than half a million Americans were incarcerated for drinking offences and consumption of illicit alcohol that contained poisonous components resulted in thousands deaths. These failures did not stop different US presidents from calling on repeated occasions for the "wars against drugs". The 1986 report of the Commission on Organized Crime admitted that America's war on drugs was not even close to success, and recommended to open the war against drug users. Mill's theory on individual freedom serves as a test against which different drug policies, their successes and failures, are tested. Taken that the drug consumption cannot be eliminated, the successful policies should focus around the risks to those who take drugs.

Legalization of some drugs with the growing taxation of them might be only one of the effective alternatives.

One of the most comprehensive and systematic works dealing with the relationship between the individual and the society in which they live is John Stuart Mill's essay *On Liberty*. It was Mill's thesis that individual liberty was the primary principle which should govern relations between the individual and society, and that there were large and important areas of human conduct which should be beyond the control of the state. Mill was worried by the tendency of the state, like some malign octopus, to take over more and more of the individual's freedom of action.

> The disposition of mankind, whether as rulers or as fellow citizens, to impose their own opinions and inclinations as a rule of conduct on others is so energetically supported by some of the best and by some of the worst feelings incident to human nature that it is hardly ever kept under restraint by anything but want of power; and as the power is not declining, but growing, unless a strong barrier of moral conviction call be raised against the mischief, we must expect, in the present circumstances of the world, to see it increase.

Mill felt that "The only purpose for which power can be rightfully exercised over any member of a civilised community, against his will, is to prevent to others. His own good, either physical or moral, is not a sufficient warrant."

Things have changed since Mill's essay was first published in 1859. As he feared, the state has increased the extent of its influence and control over the individual. Some of the legislation and government intervention has sought to promote economic security or material welfare or racial equality; and, while some might find fault with this, most of us would not. On the other hand, there are more doubtful areas in which the state has tried to exert its influence over individuals ill matters affecting their moral welfare, such as sexual practices, pornography, obscenity and, of course, the use of drugs.

National drug control policy in Britain, in the USA, and in almost all other countries is heavily committed to a model of prohibition backed by punishment. The National Drug Control Strategy for the United States in 1999 allocated two-thirds of the entire annual federal drug control budget to supply reduction measures. In 1999, the sum provided by the federal goveriiment for drug control was just under $18 billion. This was backed up by a further expenditure of about 70-80 per cent of the tens of billions of extra dollars spent on drug control by state and local governments. All of this goes towards policing, prosecution and punishment of illicit drug users. The amount to be spent from the federal allocation during 1999 on domestic law enforcement measures alone was a staggering $9 billion (about half of the entire budget). The amount allocated in 1999 to treatment (one of the only areas in which there is strong scientific evidence of effectiveness) was just over $3 billion (about one-sixth of the budget). And in stark contrast to the money freely spent on supply reduction measures, any money which is spent on treatment is linked to strict requirements to demonstrate both effectiveness and cost-effectiveness. Money is poured down the bottomless drain of prohibition, There are few points of general agreement with respect to the control of drugs. But one thing which should no longer be in doubt is that laws do not stop the use of drugs.

The earliest record of prohibitionist thought can probably be credited to an Egyptian priest who in 2000 BC, wrote: 'I, thy superior, forbid thee to go to the taverns. Thou art degraded like the beasts.' By the 16th century, a German prince was offering financial rewards to anyone who gave information leading to the conviction of coffee drinkers; and a century later, the czar of Russia executed anyone round in possession of tobacco.

In Britain during the First World War, Lloyd George laid the basis for the British system of "opening hours." Lloyd George felt that one of the most serious obstacles to increasing the output of

munitions was heavy drinking by the workforce. The factory owners who made so much profit out of the war were in complete agreement with this opinion. The Ship Building Employers Federation
asked for the closure of all public houses and clubs in the area of
any munitions factory. The king himself offered to give up alcoholic drink if it would provide an example to the workers. This ges-
ture, which became known as "The Kings Pledge," was not a success, partly, one feels, because of a conspicuous unwillingness on
the part of certain politicians and other public figures to adopt such
extreme measures. After trying various other ideas, Lloyd George
produced the Defence of the Realm Act. This drastically reduced
the availability of alcohol, and introduced the British system of
opening hours.

Whether as a result of this or of other factors, there was an
immediate and dramatic change in the nation's drinking habits
during the war. Between 1914 and 1918, the consumption of spirits was reduced by half, and that of beer was cut even more drastically, from 1,200 million gallons to 460 million gallons.
Drunkenness convictions were reduced by almost 80 per cent and
death from liver cirrhosis dropped by more than 60 per cent. For
various reasons, these changes seemed to occur mainly in the large
towns and cities; the new licensing regulations had little effect on
country areas. It is also apparent that what effects the new laws did
have were short-lived. Within a year or two, the initial effects seem
to have been swamped by other more important changes that were
taking place at the time. Quite apart from the massive social dis-
ruption that was a result of the war and the post-war economic
depression, there was already a clear national trend towards
reduced consumption of alcohol prior to the war.

This British system of control was primarily geared to restricting
the overall levels of alcohol consumption. It does not prevent
(indeed it may even encourage) "binge drinking" during the licensing hours. As closing time approaches in the British pub, it is fairly typical to find an increased tempo of drinking and an increased
number of drunks, with all that that entails.

The most dramatic efforts to control alcohol, however, have attempted to prevent any use of it. Finland and Norway have both tried this approach. Both subsequently abandoned it when it failed. But the best-known example of prohibition occurred in America between 1920 and 1933. During this period, America provided a convincing demonstration of what can go wrong with efforts to legislate drug taking out of existence.

Among the pressure groups which worked to achieve the Act of Prohibition were the temperance societies. Variously appalled both by drinking as a form of pleasure in its own right and by the wide range of social ills that they attributed to the effects of drink, they were firmly convinced that alcohol itself was sinful; and they were determined to enforce their beliefs on the rest of American society. To this end, they applied their considerable political influence.

As in Britain, part of the rationale behind the American legislation was also linked to the war effort. The Anti-Saloon League declared alcohol to be "un-American, pro-German, youth corrupting, and treasonable." The Eighteenth Amendment (otherwise known as the War Prohibition Law) was introduced partly to prevent the alcoholic subversion of the war effort, though by the time it was introduced the war had been over for a year. It attempted to remove alcohol from the American culture without providing any alternative form of satisfaction. The legislators were strong in their moral certainty that alcohol was a bad thing, but weak in their psychology. Drug taking should not be regarded merely as some trivial fault in human behaviour that can be easily corrected. Those whose business it is to pass our laws are deluding themselves if they believe that a law can achieve things that people themselves cannot.

The weight of public opinion was not behind Prohibition. Throughout the country, illicit alcohol was produced and distributed to meet the popular demand. It has been estimated that, during a one-year period, the citizens of America consumed 200 million gallons of malt liquor and 118 million gallons of wine. By 1930, more than hal a million Americans been arrested for drink offences and sentenced to a total of more than 33,000 years' imprisonment. More than a quarter of a million stills were confiscated, but the bootleg liquor continued to flow. The black market that was necessary for file manufacture and supply of illegal alcohol encouraged the involvement of organized crime: there were more than 700 gangland assassinations during Prohibition. At the same time, many public officials showed an obvious disregard for the prohibition law. Respected public figures, including many politicians in Washington, routinely broke the alcohol laws. Al Capone commented on this state of affairs:

> I make my money by supplying a public demand. If I break the law, my customers, who number hundreds of the best people in Chicago, are as guilty as I am. The only difference between us is that I sell and they buy. Everybody calls me a racketeer. I call myself a businessman. When I sell liquor, it's bootlegging. When my patrons serve it on a silver tray on Lake Shore Drive, it's hospitality.

As with other attempts to prohibit a particular drug, the black-market alternatives are frequently of poor quality. Some of the illegal alcohol that was manufactured may have been as good as the original product; some of it can only be regarded as poisonous. The consumption of illicit alcohol was responsible for 35,000 deaths, and many more were permanently incapacitated. Such was the deterrent effect of Prohibition that, in Chicago, deaths related to the use of alcohol rose by 600 per cent during that period.

Prohibition is still with us. It no longer applies to alcohol in Western societies, but to drugs; and most people accept this as a completely natural and desirable state of affairs. As with the prohibition of alcohol, the laws prohibiting drugs were passed, not so much on the basis of reasoned argument or scientific evidence, but more often as the result of some moral crusade. It is not so long since heroin, LSD, cannabis and the amphetamines were all legally available. In America, heroin and the opiates were outlawed at the same time as alcohol.

At the end of the 19th century, American newspapers "discovered" a new scandal. Lurid tales of crime and debauchery emerged, all centered on the sinister oriental menace of the opium den. Anti-Chinese feeling, which had been endemic in America throughout much of its history, was translated into a fear and hatred of one of the most characteristic habits of this group, opium smoking. Feeling at this time reached a peak of hysteria culminating in the Harrison Act. This made it impossible for the hundreds of thousands of opiates addicts in America to go on obtaining their drugs by legal means. The people who were dependent upon opiates were appalled. They wrote to the Treasury Department in the thousands, asking for "registration permits," but no such permits were available. In 1918, a number of clinics were opened to treat the addicts. Within a year the government had forced them all to close down. The addict was forced to become a criminal and associate with criminals if they wanted to go on using drugs. As a result, the myth that all addicts were criminals became a self-fulfilling prophecy: the laws had made it a criminal offence simply to be a heroin addict.

The British approach to this issue was less harsh. Throughout most of the 19th century, opiates had been freely available, and there is little evidence that this led to any dramatic increase in either the amount of the drug that was consumed or the rate of deaths from opiates. As laws were introduced to restrict the availability of specific preparations of these drugs, the public switched to other, unrestricted, forms. The influence of the recently passed Harrison Act, and the increasing pressure applied by the medical profession to limit this form of self-medication, furthered the trend towards legal control. If any final impetus was needed, it conveniently appeared in the form of scared stories about the use of morphine and cocaine by Allied troops. (This was during the most severe period of the First World War.) The use of cocaine by soldiers on leave in the West End of London was rumored to have reached alarming proportions. Respectable London stores (including Harrods) been fined for selling morphine and cocaine to the troops: one store advertised them as a "useful present for friends at the front."

These and other incidents were inflated by fears about the potential threat that such drugs might pose to national security, and they too were prohibited under the Defense of the Realm Act. In *The Lancet*, Sir William Collins confidently but mistakenly predicted that the new laws would eliminate the use of these drugs.

There is a widespread belief in the existence of a thing called "The British System" which has been applied to control the heroin problem in the UK. Belief in "The British System" tends to become stronger with increasing distance from the UK. This is often, and quite falsely, described as consisting of the widespread medical prescription of heroin to addicts. In fact, heroin was only ever used in this way during the first half of the 20th century when a very small number of (mainly middle-class and medical) addicts was provided with heroin prescriptions by private and family doctors. Since the radical changes during the 1960s, and with the vastly increased numbers of opiate addicts since that time, heroin has only rarely been made available to addicts on prescription. Current estimates suggest that there may be up to 150,000 heroin users in the UK. Only about 1 percent of these are receiving, any sort of injectable drug and only a small proportion of those are receiving a prescription for heroin. In 1990, the total number of addicts receiving injectable heroin was approximately 200. Even though this practice receives a disproportionate amount of international attention, the prescribing of heroin or other injectable drugs is numerically of small significance within the overall British response. It was largely for this reason that John String and I decided to publish our book on ' "The British System" in which Marcus Grant notes that: 'Like another British phenomenon, the, Loch Ness Monster, it is more talked about than observed and better known for its mythic dimensions than for its clear authenticity.' The latest round of the 'wars against drugs' was first declared by President Nixon in 1971, by President Ford in 1976, by President Reagan in 1982 by other drug warriors on repeated occasions since then. The war was originally intended to be a war against supply. Gradually, it turned into a real war involving the US Customs

Service, Coast Guard, Boarder Patrol, Department of Defense, Federal Aviation Administration, the intelligence agencies and even NASA. National Security Agency satellites tracked shipments of chemicals to processing laboratories in South American countries. American military teams went into the front lines in foreign countries where they destroyed coca crops and cocaine-manufacturing laboratories. Drug Enforcement Agency personnel went off to do their work in more than 40 foreign countries. Many people were assassinated or put on hit lists.

In 1986, President Regan's Commission on Organized Crime reviewed the progress of the war on drugs. The conclusion was obvious: "Despite continuing expressions of determination, America's war on drugs seems nowhere close to success." The Commission's report noted that, after three-quarters of a century of federal effort to reduce drugs supplies, there had been no reduction in the social, economic or criminal problems related to drugs. The conclusion that was drawn was that the war should be redirected against demand against the drug users themselves. Now there would be "zero tolerance" for drug takers. One anti-drugs video showed an egg ("your brain"), a simmering frying pan ("this is drugs") and a fried egg ("this is your brain on drugs"). An anti-drug poster offered advice for employers: "Help an Addict. Threaten to Fire Him." Demands were made for compulsory testing for drugs through the screening of blood or urine samples. But despite the war against drugs and drug users, drug taking continued.

Where there is a demand for drugs, prohibition does not work. It does not work whether it is alcohol, tobacco, cannabis or heroin that is being forbidden. But worse than that, it is too often forgotten that any law has certain market social costs which must be endured by society. The most serious of these is that the drug prohibition laws encourage and maintain a black market economy and a criminal subculture. Prohibition may actually increase the likelihood that those who continue to take drugs will be damaged by them either as a result of the impurities and adulterants that are sold with street drugs, or because the user who has suffered physical or psychological harm is afraid to seek help because of the illegality of drug taking. Anti-drug laws may lead otherwise law-abiding citizens into direct confrontation with the police, as a result of which they may suffer considerable social harm. Many students who have been caught experimenting with drugs have been expelled from universities and people have been dismissed from their jobs after a drug conviction. Nor are the police themselves left untouched by the prohibition laws. There have been various cases over the past few years in which members of police drug squads have been convicted on corruption charges after accepting bribes and even reselling confiscated black-market drugs. Society pays a heavy price for retaining these laws, yet there is a surprising reluctance to take account of these costs.

There were 86,000 drug seizures by police or Customs in the UK during 1993 (it is usually estimated that these represent 10 per cent or less of the total). During the same year nearly 5,000 people were imprisoned for drugs offences, almost one-third of whom were serving sentences of two years or more. Despite the trend in many countries towards increased tolerance of cannabis use, a vast amount of time, money and other resources in the UK continues to be directed towards cannabis, with more than 80 per cent of all drugs offences being related to this drug. More than 50,000 people were arrested for and convicted of unlawful possession of cannabis during 1993.

In the USA, where the War Against Drugs has been fought more intently, the unforeseen consequences of using the law to regulate drug use are greater. The anti-drug laws have been made increasingly strict. In 1993 more than 1.1 million people were arrested for drug law offences and the increase in the number of people arrested for drugs offences is directly related to the growth of the prison population. Between 1986 and 1991, the proportion of people in American prisons for drugs offences more than doubled, from less than 9 per cent to more than 21 percent. It is striking that the increase was largely due to the incarceration of black and Hispanic drug users. For black drug users, imprisonment rates increased by 447 per cent; for Hispanics, rates went up by 324 per cent. In 1994, for the first time ever, the American prison population exceeded one million. In California, which has proportionately the largest prison population in America, there are 126,000 prisoners occupying spaces intended for half that number of people. The California prison system alone costs $3 billion a year to run.

Efforts at social control do not always have predictable consequences. If architects fail so often to design successful urban living spaces, those who aspire to regulate and control our social behaviors would be well advised to show a little more humility. The efforts of police, doctors, the Pharmaceutical Association and others to restrict access to needles and syringes in Edinburgh during the early 1980s led to addicts stealing from hospital dustbins and burying injecting equipment from other users. The last retail supplier who was willing to sell injecting equipment was forced out of business in 1982, when local doctors withdrew their trade and the police put pressure on him to change his practice. This restricted access was one of the reasons for the needle sharing that led to such an explosive growth in HIV infection and hepatitis among Scottish injectors. Surveys in some areas of Scotland (notably Edinburgh and Dundee) found that up to 65 per cent of some samples of drug injectors were HIV positive. These HIV rates were as high as anywhere in the world and Edinburgh became known as the AIDS capital of Europe.

The drug prohibition laws have already established cocaine as a central part of Florida's economy. An estimated 60-80 per cent of all the cocaine that enters the USA enters through Miami: this may be more than 20 metric tons of the drug. Although this may have increased the growth rate in the standard of living by up to 5 per cent per year, the social costs, as with alcohol prohibition, include some of the worst gangland battles for many years. Local police have described their attempts to enforce cocaine prohibition laws as impossible. Whenever there is a gangland killing, or some similarly shocking episode hits the headlines, the predictable rejection is to blame the drug. In fact this crime and violence is a direct product of the prohibition laws. The organized criminal is involved because they can make huge amounts of money out of the black market. It is immaterial to them whether they deal in diamonds, paintings, illegal immigrants, heroin or alcohol. The most direct measure of the failure of the prohibition of drugs can be gauged by the fact that the international trafficking in drugs is now a business on the same scale as the international petrochemical industry or global tourism.

The Icelandic laws against alcohol are among the most strict in the Western world. The sale of beer is forbidden and alcohol is only available from state shops under very restricted conditions and at an extremely high price. There are no pubs or bars and alcohol can only be drunk publicly in restaurants. The familiar result of all this is that there is a thriving black market. Most drinkers use spirits rather than wines or beer, and, unlike the regular daily consumption of alcohol that is often found in wine-producing countries like France, the pattern of heavy drinking typically involves episodes of drunkeness followed by periods of sobriety. The Icelandic system of control is associated with one of the highest rates of alcoholism in Europe.

A different social cost of the prohibition laws lies in the waste of social resources that is involved. The Mexican government is currently directing 70 percent of its Federal Law Enforcement Budget into a campaign against the opiates, even though narcotics-related offences account for only 7 percent of the criminal prosecutions in the country. The most significant result of this is that the purity of street heroin in Mexico has dropped from 40 percent in 1976 to a mere 3 per cent. Mexican addicts are now paying more for their heroin and injecting a more impure solution into their veins.

But if prohibition of the opiates does not prevent people from using heroin, as a law it is not disregarded by any significant proportion of the population. Only a comparatively small number of people use such drugs. The laws prohibiting cannabis, however, are more questionable.

CANNABIS: THE NEW PROHIBITION

The laws that prohibit the use of drugs have not usually been con-spicuously based on scientific evidence or even on rational thought. The Eighteenth Amendment was carried onto the statute books largely as a result of the political pressure exerted by temper-ance societies; the laws against narcotics owed much to xenopho-bia (in America) and to fears about the threat to national security (in Britain). The laws against cannabis are of equally doubtful parentage.

The British laws against cannabis are almost entirely a product of the Geneva International Convention of 1925. More specifical-ly they owe a great deal to an emotional outburst by the Egyptian delegate in the discussions preceding the conference. This led to cannabis being included among the opiates and addictive drugs needing control. The British delegates were content to legislate against cannabis through their lack of interest in a drug that was hardly ever used in Europe at that time, and the Act was ratified by Parliament almost without comment.

Unlike Britain, which adopted its anti-cannabis laws more or less by default, there was no such disinterest behind the American laws. Paradoxically, the prohibition of alcohol had stimulated interest in cannabis as an alternative drug. In New York City, "tea pads" appeared. These smoking parlors were similar to opium dens, and sold cannabis very cheaply either for consumption on the premises or to take away. Such places were tolerated by the city in much the same way as the speakeasies, the illicit drinking houses, and during the early 1930s New York City alone had about 500 of them. However, the use of cannabis was not particularly wide-spread, and following the legalization of alcohol in 1933 it might well have gradually faded back into obscurity had it not been for the reawakening of interest inspired by Commissioner Anslinger.

In 1932, Harry J. Anslinger was appointed commissioner in the Federal Bureau of Narcotics. Cannabis held an intense fascination for Anslinger, who was committed to the extinction of this "lethal weed," and in his enthusiastic zeal he promoted the most misleading and ridiculous drug myths, some of which are detailed in the next chapter. But whether they were myths or not, these stories made a powerful impact both on the general public and on the legislators.

Medical authorities at the time were less impressed by the value of a further act of prohibition. One medical expert who spoke against the new bill pointed out that the case against cannabis was not based on any satisfactory scientific or medical evidence, but rested upon a few, mostly sensational, newspaper stories. And not only was the case against cannabis very weak, but there was no reason to believe that a new law would work. An editorial in the *Journal of the American Medical Association* at the time (1937, vol. 108) commented:

> The best efforts of an efficient bureau of narcotics, supplemented by the efforts of an equally efficient bureau of customs, have failed to stop the unlawful flow of opium and coca leaves and their compounds and derivatives ... What reason is there, then, for believing that any better results can be obtained by direct federal efforts to suppress a habit arising out of the misuse of such a drug as cannabis?

Other opposition was voiced by birdseed distributors who complained that canaries would not sing as well (or might even stop singing altogether!) if they were deprived of their diet of cannabis seed. Congress was sufficiently impressed by this argument to exclude sterilized cannabis seed from the bill. The opposition of the American Medical Association, on the other hand, was disregarded.

As soon as the new law had been passed, Anstinger extended his campaign against the drug. Even the medically authorized use of the drug was so energetically discouraged that it rapidly ceased altogether. Penalties against the drug increased in severity. Indeed, as recently as 1970, a first conviction for selling cannabis in Georgia could lead to a life sentence: a second conviction was punishable by death. In Louisiana, mere possession of the drug carried a minimum sentence of five years' hard labor, though the judge could sentence such vicious criminals to as much as 15 years' hard labor at their discretion. Despite the savagery of these laws, they did not stop people from using cannabis.

In most Western countries, the current trend is towards a relaxation of penalties. Many of the American states now regard possession of cannabis as a trivial offence, comparable to a minor traffic violation, In Denmark, Italy, Norway, Sweden, Switzerland, West Germany and Yugoslavia, people who have been caught in possession of small amounts of cannabis are usually let off with a warning or a small fine. Britain remains one of the few European countries that still sends people to prison for up to five years merely for possessing cannabis; only Iceland and Spain still have more severe laws. In 1992, more than 40,000 people in Britain were taken to court and convicted of cannabis-related offences (compared to 1,400 for heroin) and 1,700 people were serving prison sentences for cannabis offences (compared to 350 for heroin). The number of cannabis affects continued to climb ever upwards having increased by almost two-thirds in the five years since 1988. By 1997, the number of people convicted of cannabis offences had doubled to more than 86,000 and more than 1,900 people were in prison for cannabis offences. This seems a wasteful and misguided approach to the control of drugs.

Irrespective of how harmful cannabis may (or may not) be, this new prohibition works no better than the Eighteenth Amendment. The prohibition of alcohol produced men like Al Capone. The prohibition of cannabis has enticed organized criminals into this area and gun battles between them and the police hive been seen in America, in Europe, and now in London.

Most actions have unforeseen as well as intended consequences (as with the restriction in availability of needles in Edinburgh). The prohibition of cannabis has had many unforeseen consequences. At the personal level users have been placed in situations in which they are at greater risk of becoming involved with other, potentially more harmful, substances and patterns of use. Similar unforeseen consequences can be found at the national level.

In 1969, Operation Intercept was launched in the USA, This led to the arrest of 493 people carrying cannabis at the border with Mexico, but only small quantities of the drug were seized. Soon afterwards the name of the operation was changed to the more politically sensitive Operation Cooperation and the Mexican police were invited to destroy marijuana fields in northern Mexico. Following this, the cannabis smugglers moved further south, where they found more potent varieties of the drug. Because of the reduced supply of Mexican cannabis, other (also stronger) types were imagined from Thailand and North Africa. The average THC content of cannabis in the USA rose sevenfold as a result of these supply reduction campaigns and American consumers of the drug acquired a taste for the better quality product.

In order to meet this new demand, an industry in home-grown marijuana began to flourish in America. In 1978 the USA conducted dangerously misguided paraquat spraying programs on Mexican marijuana crops, thus providing even more incentive for domestic cultivation. One outcome was the development and cultivation of *sitisemilla,* a high-potency seedless variety of marijuana. Soon, American home-grown marijuana and its farmers had become the best in the world.

The heartland for domestic cultivation was a 10,000 square mile area of northern California – The Emerald Triangle. Indoor cultivation involving hydroponic tanks and all the latest high-tech growing halide growing lamps, methods became very popular because it was more difficult to detect. By 1987, the US home-grown marijuana crop was estimated to be worth $33.1 billion, a 150 percent increase from 1981. Supplies had gone up and demand appeared to be insatiable. By 1988, NIDA (the American National Institute on Drug Abuse) estimated that one-third of the US population aged 12 years or over (that is 66 million people) had used cannabis at least once. Anyone who wants to know how effective prohibition laws are when set against popular demand should look no further than this fact.

There are countries where the use of opium has been incorporated as a normal, or it least tolerated, social behavior. In the austere but beautiful Indian state of Rajastan, opium is quite widely used in rural areas. The drug is used in any social gatherings; it is used by men and women; its use crosses boundaries of caste and religion. In many respects, the use of opium appears to occupy the same place as alcohol in most Western countries. In such circumstances it can be extremely hazardous to introduce laws of prohibition. When this was done in Pakistan, it was almost immediately followed by the introduction of heroin powder and the rapid development of heroin smoking. Thailand had a very similar experience. In 1960, the opium prohibition law was introduced and was immediately followed by the rapid growth of a national heroin problem.

Like it or not, the tendency to use drugs would appear to be an important part of the human condition, and it is one that will not be eliminated by external restraints. Physical, fiscal and statutory means have been used at various times and in connection with various different drugs. Sometimes, they have discouraged some people from using a particular drug. Occasionally, they have failed in the most conspicuous way.

But whereas governments cannot prevent people from using certain drugs, they are capable of making it extremely convenient for people to use them. As laws of prohibition represented the least subtle means of preventing drug taking, so the Opium Wars stand as one of the least subtle examples of the promotion of drug taking.

THE OPIUM WARS

During the 18th century, England was in the grip of what the newspaper would fondly call a "drugs epidemic." The consumption of tea had increase by more than 20 times during the century, and the British government was worried about the strain imposed upon the economy by this drug which was imported mainly from China. If the Chinese had been prepared to buy British manufactured textiles there could have been an exchange of commodities between the two countries. Unfortunately, trade with foreign powers had been restricted by the Chinese government. In any case, the only commodity for which there was any demand was opium. Supposedly, this could only be imported under license, but, because of the demand for the drug, opium was smuggled into China in some quantity.

Although it is generally assumed that opium smoking has always been part of the Chinese cultural tradition it seems to have been introduced to China as late as the end of the 17th century. The commercial interest behind this was the East India Company, who cynically suggested that opium "was a pernicious article of luxury, which ought not to be permitted except for the purpose of foreign commerce." So successful was this commercial enterprise that, by the end of the 18th century, the regular use of opium was an estab-lished part of the Chinese way of life, with perhaps as many as 10 percent of the population using the drug; in some provinces the majority of the population seems to have been addicted. The unfor-tunate social effect of the drug became more widespread the abuses associated with it more unacceptable to the Chinese authorities. Opium smoking was rife among the Chinese soldiery. Out of a thousand troops sent to put down a rebellion in the province of Canton, the commanding officer was forced to reject 200 as unfit for service. When the rebels defeated the imperial forces, opium was blamed. Every part of Chinese society was affected. Three of the emperor's sons were addicts and the drug was again blamed for their deaths.

> Prohibition had been completely unsuccessful, despite the fact that it wa, reinforced by flogging, exile, imprisonment and finally death. In the end the emperor sent Imperial Comissioner Lin to Canton to suppress the illicit traffic in opium. After making various appeals to the British, including a letter which was sent to Queen Victoria (but was never delivered), Lin confiscated and destroyed almost 2,500,000 pounds of British opium. It was mixed with lime and salt, dissolved in water and flushed into the sea.

Angered by this affront to British dignity, no less than by the considerable loss of revenue involved, Lord Palmerston and the government decided that China must be compelled to pay compensation for enforcing its own laws, against smuggled drugs. It was also to be compelled to extend the British right to import opium. A naval force of 16 warships backed up by 7,000 troops was sent to enforce this arrangement, which it duly did. Imperial policy, however, remained the same in its attempt to enforce the ineffective laws against opium smuggling. In 1856, more than 10 years after Commissioner Lin's confiscation of opium in Canton, the new emperor sent another commissioner to resume Lin's policies. As a result, the *Arrow* was seized. The *Arrow* was a Chinese-owned smuggling ship which had been registered as a British vessel in Hong Kong. Again Palmerston sent out the gunboats. The commissioner's official residence was shelled, and a British expeditionary force occupied Peking and burned down the emperor's Summer Palace. As before, the military contest was one-sided, and as part of the settlement China was compelled to accept unlimited imports of opium on payment of a duty. Afterwards, there was a massive increase both in the amounts of opium imported into China and in the corresponding economic benefits to the British government.

So successful was the opium trade that, in many Asian countries, good agricultural land was turned over to the cultivation of the poppy instead of food crops. Whole communities became dependent upon the production of opium, and the local warlords found it a reliable source of revenue. During the Japanese occupation of these territories in the 1930s and 1940s, opium was used to provide revenue for the occupation forces and morphine factories were set up. Throughout Asia there are many communities that rely upon the opium crop for their survival. The same is true in a number of Middle Eastern countries where the poppy is the staple of village life. Its oil is a base for cooking, its leaves can be used to make a salad, its seeds to enrich the bread, and the pods to feed cattle. And there remains the gum itself, which can be sold to many interested parties. Once the poppy has become an established crop, it is very difficult to eradicate it. Once the opium is available, the temptations for the drug smugglers are enormous. The Opium Wars were a comparatively trivial incident in history, but their consequences are still very much with us.

ALTERNATIVE METHODS OF CONTROL

Somewhere between total prohibition (which is ineffective) and the promotion of drugs by the state (which is undesirable) there remain a number of less dramatic alternatives. These may include state rationing, state-run monopolies, restriction of outlets for the sale of drugs, licensing hours and limited forms of prohibition which may apply to children (or other stigmatized groups, possibly including women or ethnic minorities).

Undoubtedly, there is a need for better information to be made available about drugs and their effects. A better informed public might use drugs more sensibly and suffer less harm from them as a result. However, it would be naive to imagine that to provide the public with such information would necessarily lead to any dramatic decrease in drug use. Indeed, it is possible that unrealistic fears about drugs may sometimes serve as a deterrent to drug use.

The early abolitionists believed that teaching children "the evils of alcohol" would lead to abstinence, but it didn't. Since anti-drug propaganda does not prevent the use of drugs, there is little reason to expect impartial drug information to do so. Psychologists have found little evidence that knowledge and behavior are directly related. A person may know that riding a fast motorcycle is extremely dangerous and still continue to do so; equally, knowing that air travel is one of the safest forms of transport does not stop many people from being terrified of flying

A good deal of drug education has been an anxiety-stricken enterprise which has tried to "innoculate" children with "preventative" information that will keep them safe from drugs. This approach has not worked. All too often it has failed because the educational material has purveyed an alarming but completely unrealistic picture of drugs and drug taking. The "facts" have simply not been true, and they have not deterred children from experimenting with drugs. Most of the studies that have looked at the effects of drug education have found that it makes little impression upon attitudes and has had no consistent effect on subsequent behavior. For ears, health education programs have emphasized the risks associated with cigarette smoking. Cigarette packets carry government health warnings. No one who smokes can have avoided exposure to this deluge of information, yet millions of people continue puffing away.

In 1988, California increased the excise tax on a packet of cigarettes from 10 to 35 cents. Of the expected $600 million revenue, 20 percent was earmarked for health education purposes. Much of this was spent on a campaign that was designed to undermine the credibility of the tobacco industry. One anti-smoking advertisement carried the message, "Warning: the tobacco industry is not your friend."

There is an urgent need to reassess what drug education can realistically be expected to achieve. It is vital that everyone realizes that it cannot *eliminate* drug taking. What it could do is to reduce the amount of harm that people suffer as a result of their drug taking, If the quality of information about drugs was better, and if it was more widely available, it might help people to use drugs more intelligently. If the relative hazards of the different drugs were fully appreciated, those who chose to take drugs might avoid the more obviously dangerous ones.

Fortunately, attempts to direct drug prevention activities towards reducing the harm suffered by users are now, at last, gradually becoming respectable and acceptable. It is sad that it has taken something as threatening as AIDS to produce this change of direction, but at least late is better than never. There are still committed abolitionists who remain opposed to harm-reduction initiatives and who expect prevention campaigns to present drug taking as dangerous, unpleasant and totally unacceptable. For some, anything less than zero tolerance reeks of collusion.

Few of us are in favor of the individual systematically harming himself; it is, nonetheless, legally permissible to eat yourself to death, or indeed to smoke and drink yourself to death. Since the Suicide Act was passed, you can deliberately kill yourself by taking an overdose of legally available drugs or of a legally available poison. Yet we retain laws prohibiting the recreational use of certain drugs. These laws have comparatively little to do with the intrinsic dangers of the drugs involved (though this issue is always one of the first to be cited by proponents of the existing prohibition laws): for instance, the available evidence suggests that cannabis is a less harmful drug than alcohol, yet this provides little impetus towards changing the legal status of these drugs.

A more central principle in this issue is that of society seeking to protect the individual from the consequences of their own actions. This principle was first stated by Plato who argued that the state must save its citizens from the corruptions that are intrinsic to the masses; it is based upon a belief that the general public lack the intelligence, discipline and motivation to protect or even to know what is in their own interests. Unfortunately, drug taking may well be something from which people do not want to be saved.

Among the other factors behind the drug prohibition laws is the desire of certain sections of society to suppress anything that upsets or offends them. It is interesting that the Third Reich was committed to the drive against smoking and sponsored many anti-smoking campaigns. Cigarettes were banned in many public places and from Luftwaffe premises. SS officers were forbidden to smoke when on duty, and cigarette advertising which featured sportsmen, attractive women and fast cars was banned. In recent years, the view that the state has every right to ban behavior which is deemed to be offensive was vigorously expressed by Lord Devlin, who argued that the law is a legitimate means of forcing the individual to adopt conventional moral codes of conduct. Devlin's argument turns on the point that anything which offends the community may justifiably be made against the law.

John Stuart Mill had anticipated each of these paternalist arguments and found them repugnant.

So monstrous a principle is far more dangerous than any single interference with liberty; it acknowledges no right to freedom whatever, except perhaps to that of holding opinions in secret, without ever disclosing them; for the moment an opinion which I consider noxious passes anyone's lips, it invades all the social rights attributed to me.

However, the way in which we are to separate the rights of the individual and the notion of harm to others is not entirely straight-forward. Many drugs, and especially those such as tobacco and alcohol which are most widely used, impose a considerable burden upon others in society who must pick up the costs of health care and economic loss through accidents, industrial inefficiencies and so on. Although these costs are impossible to quantify with any accuracy, it is clear that they are very high. The economic costs to the USA of alcohol problems alone are estimated at over $100,000 dollars per year. In addition, there are other incalculable costs, such as the misery caused by friends or relatives being injured by drunk drivers.

We are increasingly aware of the many costs of drug taking. However, John Stuart Mill was not unaware of these issues and he did consider an alternative form of restrictions that although the state should permit such forms of behavior as drug taking which might be against the best interests of the individual, it could also indirectly discourage such behavior. One way of doing so is through taxation.

This system is already used for alcohol and tobacco, both of which have, carried a high excise duty for so long that this is accept-ed as a fact of life. (The actual cost of a bottle of whisky is only about one-fifth of its retail price.) For some years now, there has been a growing acceptance of the notion that the incidence of drug-related problems in society is closely related to the average consumption levels in that society. As a result there has developed a preference for tackling such problems by using legislative controls. The com-ments of the advisory committee to the British government in 1977 reflect a good deal of common sense in this matter:

We do not recommend, for example, that alcoholic drink should, by the increase of taxation, be priced out of the reach of many people. We consider that this step would unfairly penalize the vast majority of unaddicted drinkers, and do nothing to reduce the incidence of alcoholism amongst those who could still afford it, whilst tempting those who could not toward dangerous alternative sources of intoxication.

It is still not clear precisely how taxation does affect consumption. Detailed analyses show that, whenever there has been an increase in the cost of alcohol or tobacco, there has been a short-term fall in consumption (or the rate of consumption has increased less sharply). There seems to be some link between the price of a drug and levels of consumption, but this relationship is often rather weak. Between 1960 and 1990, there was a, steady decline in the use of tobacco in the UK. During that time, the real (inflation adjusted) price of tobacco also fell. The principal factor affecting demand during that time seems to have been, not price, but changes in attitudes towards smoking possibly related to health warnings and health education programs but more probably associated with the complex and unquantifiable shifts that occur in social belief systems over time. Similarly, in Ireland, where alcohol is expensive as a result of high taxation, this had led to a large proportion of income being devoted to the purchase of drink, rather than to any fill in consumption. Since most of the studies of the link between price and consumption have been done with the legal drugs such as alcohol and tobacco, it is unclear what sort of link might exist for other types of drugs.

If legalization or some form of state regulation of what are currently illegal drugs is ever to take place, the economic regulation of drug consumption will become important. It has often been assumed that the demand for illegal drugs is likely to be independent of the cost of the drug; that is, relatively large increases in price would leave demand unchanged (in the jargon of economists, this sort of demand is elegantly described as being "price-inelastic"). When this is the case, supply reduction efforts tend not only to be ineffective, they are also frequently counterproductive. For example, users may turn to crime to obtain money, arid tile use of adulterated drugs may increase. Heroin users switch from chasing the dragon to the more cost-efficient but more dangerous method of injecting heroin because of the high cost of their habit. At present, very little is known about the effects of price upon demand for different types of illegal drugs by users at different stages of their drug-taking careers.

In any case, there are problems involved in using taxation as a way of controlling the use of drugs which are currently only available from illicit sources. If these drugs were legally available, but taxed heavily enough to deter consumption, there would be an incentive to evade paying the tax by using the illegal channels of distribution that already exist. This problem is already evident with the growth of cigarette and tobacco smuggling which has established itself across Europe within the past decade. Conversely, if prices were reduced to sufficiently low levels to cut out any profits for black-market supply networks, there would bed risk that the low price of the drug would increase availability and increase the numbers of people who would take the drug. Other problems to be addressed in any consideration of the state regulation of drugs might include the details of how retail sales might be organized, age limits and restrictions in the circumstances in which drug taking would be permitted.

Another way in which the state can attempt to influence the consumption of drugs is through advertising. It remains an intriguing but unanswered advertising really does affect the amount of drugs that question whether people take. The companies that advertise cigarettes and alcohol have argued that advertising does not turn non-users into users, but that its major purpose is to change brand preferences. The manufacturers would like us to believe this was true. The cigarette and alcohol-control lobbies would wish us to believe otherwise. In fact, there is little evidence one way or the other. No one knows to what extent cigarette and alcohol advertising contributes toward the consumption or abuse of these drugs.

One of the few occasions on which a government has prohibited the advertising of alcohol and tobacco occurred in British Columbia from 1971 to 1972. This was done in the hope that it would reduce smoking and drinking, especially among young people. The ban proved to be generally unpopular: six months after it was introduced almost two-thirds of the population was opposed to it, and after only 12 months the ban was lifted. The Addiction Research Foundation of Toronto, which examined the effects of the ban as it related to the consumption of alcohol, found no evidence that it led to any reduction in drinking. Ultimately, the control of drug taking always remains in the hands of the individual, and the best chance of achieving effective control lies in helping each person to make a responsible choice.

DEBATE QUESTIONS:

The author, Michael Gossop, supports John Stuart Mill's conception of liberty. According to Mill, what is the only reason the government may curtail an individual's liberty? Can the government curtail an individual's liberty for his own good?

On page 124, the author writes, 'The tendency to use drugs would appear to be an important part of the human condition.' What evidence does he use to support this claim? Do you agree with him?

While, like Mill, the author does not approve of 'paternalistic' laws, he does address the issue of taxing drug use. What does he say about taxation? Do you find his argument persuasive?

NOTES

Taken from Michael Gossop, "Living with Drugs", 5th ed., Ashgate ARENA, 2000, pp 167 - 185. Used with permission.

Drug Legalization, Harm Reduction and Drug Policy[1]

Robert DuPont, Institute for Behavior and Health, Inc
& Eric Voth, The International Drug Strategy

This article takes on the prohibitionist's perspective, explaining the history of drug policy in the United States and advocates against less restrictive policies that are generally referred to as "drug legalization", the negative global experience with legal drugs such as alcohol and tobacco being the main argument. The paper concludes that only the strong national policy reducing harm through abuse prevention will be successful.

The current U.S. policy options on drug use are reviewed in the context of the history of drug policy in the United States. A restrictive drug policy is a deterrent to drug use and helps reduce drug-related costs and societal problems. Although legalization or decriminalization of drugs might reduce some of the legal consequences of drug use, increased drug use would result in harmful consequences.

Two opposing policy options shape the current debate on how to proceed in addressing the problems with drug use in the United States[2]. One school of thought, broadly labeled "prohibition," supports widening interdiction, treatment, and prevention efforts while keeping of amnesia of the tragic consequences of widespread drug drugs such as marijuana, cocaine, LSD, and heroin illegal. A conflicting viewpoint called "legalization" supports eliminating restrictive drug policy while trying to limit the harms associated with the nonmedical use of drugs[3]. An understanding of the history of drug control in United States places the current debate on drug policy in perspective.

BACKGROUND

Modern drug prohibition began in the 19th when the medicinal chemistry industry began to produce many potent and habituating drugs. One such drug was heroin, which was first sold in the United States in 1898. These drugs were sold as ordinary commercial items along with a popular new drink, cocaine-containing Coca-Cola. At that time, physicians freely prescribed addicting drugs to their patients, thereby producing a large group of medical addicts. Drugs such as cocaine were originally used for legitimate medical indications. Drug use by the public later rapidly grew to include compulsive use, illegal activity to support nonmedical use, and consumption despite clear negative medical and social consequences.

This era of indiscriminate sale and use of addictive drugs ended during the first two decades of the 20th century with a new social contract embodied in the Pure Food and Drug Act of 1906[4], which addressed the labeling of drugs. In 1914, the Harrison Narcotics Act[5] prohibited the sale of narcotics. The Voistead Act, along with the 18th Amendment to the Constitution in 1919, prohibited the sale of alcohol. These laws were part of a broad reform movement in the United States that also promoted women's right to vote.

Under this new social contract, habituating drugs were not available except through a physician's prescription; even then the drugs were used sparingly in treating illnesses other than addiction. In 1933, alcohol was removed from the list of strictly controlled or prohibited substances. In 1937, marijuana was added to the list of prohibited substances because of a sudden increase in the use of the drug[6]. The patent drug epidemic had begun with morphine and heroin in the final decade of the 19th century and ended with an explosive increase in the use of cocaine during the first decade of the 20th century.

The social contract regulating drugs of abuse served the country well by nearly ending the first drug abuse epidemic The U.S. drug control laws proved to be a model throughout the world during the first two thirds of the 20th century. The use of habituating drugs, which been out of control at the end of the 19th century, was dramatically reduced in the United States between 1920 and 1965[6].

The nation was lulled into complacency by the great and prolonged success of this drug abuse policy. Public and policy leaders in the United States entered a period of amnesia of the tragic consequences of widespread drug use. By the 1960s, most Americans had no personal memory of the earlier U.S. addiction epidemic. Strict prohibition of nonalcohol drugs was broadly respected until the ascendant youth culture integrated drugs as a central the element of its new lifestyles.

Marijuana, the hallucinogens, and cocaine became option widely defined as "marginally addictive" or "soft" drugs[7]. Their use became the focus of a call for legalization based on unsubstantiated claims that these drugs were no worse than alcohol and tobacco. Both the substantial century health and addictions problems now known to result from the use of crack cocaine and marijuana and the extensive research on the harmful effects of many drugs are testimony to the manner in which society was misled in the 1960s[8]. These effects include addiction, vehicular trauma, disease, suicide, and specific negative physical effects of the drugs themselves[9-16].

LEGALIZATION OF ILLEGAL DRUGS

In recent years, the drug legalization movement has gained modest public support by attempting to associate opponents of drug legalization with the negative public perceptions of alcohol prohibition and by calling the opponents of legalization prohibitionists. For this discussion, we define prohibition as a restrictive policy that maintains legal restrictions against the nonmedical use or sale of addicting drugs, as covered under the Controlled Substances Act[17].

TABLE 1. DRUG USE IN THE UNITED STATES*

Variable	Year 1985	1993	Decrease in Use %
	nT		
Drugs legal for adults			
Alcohol	113	103	9
Cigarettes	60	50	17
Most widely used drugs illegal for all ages			
Marijuana	18	9	50
Cocaine	6	1.3	78

Adapted from reference 20. T Values refer to the number (in millions) of persons using the listed drugs. Data reflect use in a 30-day period.

Drug legalization is neither a simple nor singular public policy proposal. For example, drug legalization could at one extreme involve a return to open access to all drugs for all persons, as was seen at the end of the 19th century. Partial legalization could entail such policy changes as making currently illegal drugs available in their crude forms to certain types of ill patients. This limited legalization might include the maintenance of persons addicted to heroin or their drug of choice, distribution of needles to addicts without requiring that they stop using drugs, or marked softening of sentencing guidelines for drug-related offenses.

The evidence of the negative global experience with the legal substances tobacco and alcohol is overlooked by most supporters of drug legalization. The data on alcohol and tobacco support the view that legalization of drugs leads to large increases in the use of the legalized drugs and to higher total social costs. These added costs are primarily paid in lost productivity, illness, and death. In the United States, about 125 000 and 420 000 deaths are annually attributed to alcohol and tobacco, respectively. Fewer than 10 000 deaths each year result from the use of all illicit drugs combined. The social costs from alcohol use in the United States are estimated to be $86 billion, whereas the annual costs of prohibiting illegal drug use (including enforcement and incarceration) are $58 billion[18, 19]. The social costs of tobacco use are estimated to be $65 billion annually[18]. If one of the goals of a drug policy is to reduce the harm to society that results from drug use, then alcohol and tobacco must be a top priority within this strategy.

Considering the number of users of illegal and legal drugs in the United States and the trends in the rates of use from 1985 to 1991 (Table 1), it becomes apparent that prohibitive drug policy has actually maintained low levels of use compared with the wide availability of habituating substances. Equally important are the rates of illicit drug use, which have decreased faster than the rates of legal drug use[20].

Substantial progress was made in reducing adolescent drug use from 1978 to 1992 (Table 2). That success was due to a relatively clear national message and broadbased antidrug efforts in both the public and private sectors. Since 1992, adolescent drug use has increased, and attitudes toward drug use have become more accepting[21]. Although these changes have many causes, the reduction of government and media antidrug efforts and increases in media campaigns promoting drugs have played a role.

HARM REDUCTION

Although reducing the harm caused by drug use is a universal goal of all drug policies, policy proposals called "harm reduction" proposals include a creative renaming of the dismantling of legal restrictions against the use and sale of drugs. The essential components of legalization policies are couched within this concept. Much of the driving force behind the harm reduction movement also centers on personal choice and "safe" habits for drug use[22].

Paradoxically, some public policy attempts at reducing the harms associated with the use of alcohol and tobacco involve tightening restrictions on intoxicated driver legislation and smoking restrictions[23], whereas current harm reduction proposals generally involve softening the restrictions on the use of illegal drugs.

The current harm reduction proposals for drugs other than tobacco or alcohol focus heavily on reducing or eliminating criminal penalties for drug offenses, softening sentencing guidelines, providing addict maintenance programs and needle exchange programs for intravenous drug users, and removing work-place drug testing programs[24]. The efficacy of these proposals has not been established.

As it is represented in the current policy debate, harm reduction policy also attempts to mitigate the negative effects of nonmedical drug use without reducing the use of illegal drugs. The policy is based on the assumption that most of the harm caused by nonmedical drug use is the result of the societal efforts to stop drug use rather than the result of drug use itself. Those harms are generally considered to be associated with arrests from and legal consequences of illegal behavior and with incarceration[25]. Advocates of harm reduction contend that essentially innocent drug users are targeted by prohibition; however, only 2% of federal inmates are incarcerated for possession-related crime compared with 48% incarcerated for drug trafficking. Despite the clear deterring effect of legal penalties, some positive outcomes can be attributed to the criminal justice system. For example, 35% of persons imprisoned for drug-related offenses are treated for drug addiction while incarcerated[26].

In the Netherlands, an international model for decriminalization and harm reduction, decriminalization has been associated with an increase in crime and drug use.

TABLE 2. RATES OF MARIJUANA USE IN HIGH SCHOOL SENIORS*

Frequency of Use	Year							
	1978	1986	1987	1988	1991	1992	1993	1994
				%-				
Last 12 months	50.2	39	36	33.1	23.9	21.9	26	30.7
Last 30 Days	37.1	23.4	21	18	13.8	11.9	15.5	19
Daily	10.7	4.0	3.3	2.7	2.0	1.9	2.4	3.6

Adapted from reference 20.

From 1984 to 1992, cannabis use among students in the Netherlands increased 250%. Between 1988 and 1993, the number of registered addicts increased 22%. Also reflecting the decriminalization of marijuana, the number of marijuana addicts increased 30% from 1991 to 1993 alone. As we see in the United States, the harms of increased drug use go beyond those to the user alone. Since the tolerant drug policy was instituted in the Netherlands, shootings have increased 40%, hold-ups have increased 69%, and car thefts have increased 62% (Gunning KF. Personal communication).

In the United States, we experimented briefly with the decriminalization of marijuana. That temporary softening of drug policy resulted in a statistically significant increase in the reported number of marijuana-related visits to emergency departments compared with metropolitan areas in which marijuana use was not decriminalized[27].

The current and still dominant drug policy seeks to curb drug use and the associated harms by using the legal system and other methods such as work-place drug testing and treatment to reduce nonmedical drug use. In contrast to the advocates of harm reduction or legalization, supporters of the current restrictive drug policy emphasize that most drug-related harm is caused by drug use and not just by drug prohibition[28].

The two groups find some common ground in the support of drug education and treatment. Supporters of restrictive drug policy teach complete avoidance of nonmedical drug use, and harm reductionists support teaching "responsible use" of currently illegal drugs. Many proponents of harm reduction admit that they seek the ultimate legalization of illegal drugs, especially marijuana. Some harm reduction supporters advocate this policy because decriminalization would relieve the legal pressure on their own drug use. These persons seek to manipulate drug policy to justify their own drug-using behaviors.

Clearly, all forms of legalization, including harm reduction, are strategies ultimately aimed at softening public and government attitudes against nonmedical drug use and the availability of currently illegal drugs.

COSTS OF DRUG POLICY

Advocates of legalization correctly point out that prohibiting the use of our currently illegal drugs is expensive. The sources of overall costs produced by the use of legal drugs compared with costs of illegal drug use are listed in Table 3. These data also show that restrictive drug policy shifts the costs of drug use related to health and productivity to the criminal justice system.

Augmenting a restrictive drug policy by broadening the drug treatment available to addicts may be beneficial and cost-effective. A recent study by RAND[29] estimates that the current societal costs and actual costs of controlling cocaine use alone total $42 billion annually ($13 billion for control costs and $29 for societal costs).

This study also estimated that the net control and societal costs related to cocaine could be reduced to $33.9 billion by maintaining our current enforcement policies and adding to it the treatment of all addicts. The RAND study concluded that the treatment is effective in reducing the costs to society not only by reducing the demand for drugs but also by removing the addict from drugs for sustained periods of time.

TABLE 3. ECONOMIC COSTS OF ADDICTION IN THE UNITED STATES IN 1990*

Variable	Illicit Drugs	Alcohol	Tobacco
Total cost, $	66.9	98.6	72
Medical care, $	3.2 (4.8)	10.5 (10.7)	20.2 (28)
Lost productivity, $	8.0 (11.9)	36.6 (37.1)	6.8 (9.0)
Death, $	3.4 (5.1)	33.6 (34.1)	45 (63.0)
Crime, $	46.0 (68.8)	15.8 (16.0)	0.0 (0.0)
Acquired immunodeficiency syndrome, $	6.3 (9.4)	2.1 (2.1)	0.0 (0.0)

Adapted from reference 17. Costs are expressed as billions of dollars.

Supporters of restrictive drug policy must acknowledge that prohibition alone does not eliminate either the use of prohibited drugs or the high cost to society that results from the use of these drugs. Furthermore, drug prohibition achieves its goals at a substantial cost in the form of maintaining the criminal justice system and restricting personal choice. Prohibiting the use of some drugs is undeniably costly; however, because the overall level and total societal costs of drug use are reduced, this prohibition is well worth the cost.

DRUG POLICY OPTIONS

Given the range of options available within legalization and drug prohibition policies, it is important to look at the overall picture of drug policy. We must ask whether prohibiting the consumption of some drugs is effective in reducing social costs, or "harm," and whether restrictive policy is cost-effective. Two models for drug policy help answer these questions.

The first model examines life in the United States 100 years ago, a time when habituating drugs were sold like toothpaste or candy. At the end of the 19th century, Americans considered the problems with freely available habituating drugs unacceptable. In the context of today's debate on drug policy, it should be recalled that prohibition policies resulted from a nonpartisan outcry over the serious negative effects of uncontrolled drug use. In other words, the prohibition of marijuana, heroin, and cocaine did not cause widespread drug use in the United States. Rather, widespread use of those drugs use caused their prohibition. Furthermore, prohibition of nonalcohol drugs was successful in reducing drug use and was almost universally supported by all political parties in the United States and throughout the world for half a century.

While it lasted, alcohol prohibition was also largely successful from a health perspective. For example, the number of deaths from cirrhosis of the liver decreased from 29.5/100000 persons in 1911 to 10.7/100000 persons in 1929. Admissions to state mental hospitals for alcohol psychosis decreased from 10/100000 persons in 1919 to 4.7/100000 persons in 1928[30]. The main failure of alcohol prohibition was its attempt to remove the availability of alcohol from the public after it had been legal, accepted, and deeply integrated into society for many years. Currently illegal drugs do not share that same level of acceptance and integration.

The second model for drug policy compares the costs generated by the drugs that are now legal for adults with the costs of those that are not. This entails comparing the social costs resulting from the use of alcohol and tobacco (legal drugs) with costs of using marijuana, cocaine, heroin, and other illegal drugs. Alcohol and tobacco produce more harm than all of the illegal drugs combined because they are so widely used, and they are more widely used because they are legal. As legal substances, they enjoy greater social acceptance, widespread advertising, and glorification. The national experience with alcohol and tobacco does not represent an attractive alternative to the prohibition of drug use as it is currently practiced in the United States and other countries.

TABLE 4. PREVALENCE OF DRUG USE IN U.S. HIGH SCHOOL SENIORS, 1993*

Drug	Lifetime Use	Last 30 Days
	%	%
Any illicit drug	43	18
Marijuana	35	16
Cocaine	6	1.3
Alcohol	87	51
Cigarettes	62	30

Adapted from reference 20

Because alcohol and tobacco are deeply integrated into society, prohibiting their use is politically unrealistic. However, major constraints on the use alcohol and tobacco, such as total elimination of advertising, high taxation, restriction on smoking locations, designated driver programs, and product liability by the manufacturers and distributors of these products, show some promise in reducing the harm produced by these legal drugs[24].

RECOMMENDATIONS

The relevant policy question is whether legalization or reducing the restrictions on the availability of drugs would increase the number of drug users and total social bar produced by the use of currently illegal drugs. The available data show that legalization would increase the use of currently prohibited drugs[4, 21, 28].

Legalization or decriminalization creates a particular risk among young persons whose social adaptation and maturation are not yet Complete. This fact can be shown by comparing the levels of the use of currently legal drugs by young persons (alcohol and tobacco) with the levels of illegal drug use. The use of all of these drugs is illegal for young persons, but the drugs that are legal for adults are more widely used by youths than the drugs that are illegal for both adults and young persons (Table 4).

What is needed today is not the dismantling of restrictive drug policies. Rather, a strong national policy should seek to reduce the harm of drug use through harm prevention (for example, by creating drug-prevention programs) and harm elimination (by implementing broader interdiction and rehabilitation efforts)[31-33]. This new policy should strengthen efforts to reduce the use of alcohol and tobacco as well as currently illegal drugs. In so doing, this policy should take aim at especially vulnerable persons in the community, with a special emphasis on the young.

If persons who seek to reform drug policy and harm reduction are sincere in their intent, they would focus their efforts on alcohol and tobacco, substances for which "harm reduction" is greatly needed, and leave the currently illegal drugs illegal. Unless those who subscribe to the notion of harm reduction move ahead to prevention and elimination of harm, the global costs associated with any form of drug use will continue to increase. Relaxation of the restrictive policies on the use of currently illegal drugs should only be considered in the context of programs that can first prove drastic and lasting reductions in alcohol and tobacco use. Real harm reduction involves prohibiting illegal drugs while concurrently working to prevent and treat their use. We do not need new experiments to tell us what we have already learned from legal alcohol and tobacco. Those experiments have already been done at the cost of great human suffering.

NOTES

[1] Taken from Annals of Internal Medicine, 1995 123: 461-465
[2] De Leone G. Some problems with the anti-prohibitionist position on legalization of drugs. J. Addict Dis., 1994; 13:35-57
[3] U.S. General Accounting Office, General Government Division. Confronting the drug problem-debate persists on enforcement and alternative

approaches. GAO/GGD-93-82. Report to the Chairman, Committee on Government Operations, House of Representatives. Washington, DC: United States General Accounting Office, General Government Division; 1993.

4 Pure Food and Drug Act of 1906. Public Law 59-384.

5 Harrison Narcotics Act. Public Law 63-47.

6 Musto DF. The American Disease: Origins of Narcotic Control. New York: Oxford Univ Pr; 1987.

7 Brecher EM. Licit and Illicit drugs. Boston: Little, Brown; 1972: 267-306, 335-451.

8 U.S. Department of Health and Human Services. Drug Abuse and Drug Abuse Research: The Third Triennial Report to Congress from the Secretary, Department of Health and Human Services. DHHS Publication no. (ADM) 91-1704. Washington, DC: U.S. Government Pr,,ntng Office; 1991.

9 Be an AL, Schwartz RH. Suicide @ittempts among adolescent drug users. Am J Dis Child. 1990;144:310-4.

10 Rivara FP, Mueller BA, Fligner CL, Luna G, Raisys VA, Copass M, et a]. Drug use in trauma victims. J Trauma. 1989;29:462-70.

11 Soderstrom CA, Dischinger PC, Smith GS, McDuff DR, Hebei JR, Gorelick DA. Psychoactive substance dependence among trauma center patients. JAMA. 1992;267:2756-9.

12 Committee on Drug Abuse of the Council on Psychiatric Services. Position statement on psychoactive substance use and dependence: update on marijuana and cocaine. Am J Psychiatry. 1987;144:698-702.

13 Polen MR, Sidney S, Tekawa IS, Sadler M, Friedman GD. Health care use by frequent marijuana smokers who do not smoke tobacco. West J Med. 1993;158:596-601.

14 Nahas G, Latour C. The human toxicity of marijuana. Med J Aust. 1992;156:495-7.

15 Schwartz RH. Marijuana: an overview. Pediatr Clin North Am. 1987; 34:305-17

16 Mariiuana: its health hazards and therapeutic potentials. Council on Scientific Affairs. JAMA. 1981;246:1823-7.

17 Controlled Substances Act of 1970. 21 U.S.C. 811.

18 Horgan CM. Institute for Health Policy, Brandeis University. Substance Abuse: The Nation's Number One Health Problem-Key Indicators for Policy. Princeton, NJ: Robert Wood Johnson Foundation; 1993.

19 U.S. Department ofjustice, Bureau ofjustice Statistics. The costs of illegal drug use. In: Drugs, Crime, and the Criminal Justice System. NCJ-133652, 126-127. Washington, DC: U.S. Department of Justice, Bureau of Justice Statistics; 1992.

20 *National Institute on Drug Abuse. National Household Survey on Drug Abuse: Main Findings. DHHS Publication No. (SMA) 93-1980. Rockville, MD: U.S. Department of Health and Human Services, Substance Abuse and Mental Health Services Administration, Office of Applied Studies; 1993.*

21 U.S. Department of Health and Human Services, Public Health Service, National Institutes of Health. National Survey Results on Drug Use from the Monitoring the Future Study 1975-1993. NIH Publication No. 94-3809.

Rockville, MD: U.S. Department of Health and Human Services; 1994.

[22] Erickson PG. Prospects of harm reduction for psychostimulants. In: Heather N, ed. Psychoactive Drugs and Harm Reduction: From Faithto Science. London: Whurr; 1993:196.

[23] Gostin LO, Brandt AM. Criteria for evaluating a ban on the advertisement of cigarettes. Balancing public health benefits with constitutional burdens. JAMA 1993;269:904-9

[24] Nadelman E, Cohen P, Locher U, Stimson G, Wodak A, Drucker E. Position paper on harm reduction. In: The Harm Reduction Approach to Drug Control: International Progress. New York: The Lindesmith   Center; 1994.

[25] Kleiman MA. The drug problem and drug policy: what have we learned from the past four years. Testimony to the U.S. Senate Committee of the Judiciary; 29 April 1999

[26] Maguire K, ed. Sourcebook of Criminal Statistics Bureau of Justice Statistics. Washington, DC: U.S. Department of Justice; 1992:491.

[27] Model KE. The effect of marijuana decriminalization on hospital emergency room drug episodes: 1975-1978. Journal of the American Statistical Association. 1993;88:737-47

[28] Kleber HD. Our current approach to drug abuse-progress, problems, N Engl J Med. 1994;330:361-5.

[29] Rydell CP, Everingbam SS. Controlling Cocaine: Supply Versus Demand Programs. Santa Monica, CA.: RAND; 1994

[30] Gold MS. The Good News about Drugs and Alcohol. New York:Villard Books; 1991:245.

[31] Drug abuse in the United States. Strategies for prevention. JAMA. 1991;265:2102-7.

[32] Romer D. Using mass media to reduce adolescent involvement in drug trafficking. Pediatrics. 1994;93:1073-7

[33] Voth E. The war on drugs: time to relocate the battlefield? [Letter]. JAMA. 1995;273:459.

DEBATE QUESTIONS:

Whereas the thrust of Gossop's article was philosophical –
drugs should be legalized because people should be free to use
them – Dupont and Voth's argument is based on questions of
policy. According to these authors does drug legalization
increase or decrease drug use?

The authors point to the example of the Netherlands. What
does that example show? Also, would these authors agree
that private behavior should be left private because it does
not have any bearing on the public?

Do you agree that 'the relevant policy question is whether
legalization or reducing the restrictions on the availability of
drugs would increase the drug users and total social harm
produced by the use of currently illegal drugs'? What else
might be the 'relevant policy question'? What do you think
Gossop might say?

To Take Arms Against the Sea of Drugs[1]

Dr Alex Wodak
Director, Alcohol and Drug Service,
St Vincent's Hospital, New South Wales, Australia

Different arguments for and against restrictive drug policies can be presented in different ways, depending on the point of view of the presenter. This is why it is difficult to come up with the true meaning of some terms. What do we mean when we say "legalization"? Is it uncontrollable availability of substances that were considered to be illicit on the market, or should there be any control over them? What are the alternatives to supply reduction policies and may be they are too many to efficiently chose from? Controlled availability of current illicit substances emerges as an answer to these questions.

Restricting availability is the major response to illicit drugs globally and has been adopted in almost all countries. The health, social, and economic costs of supply reductions, however, are substantial and are increasing for both injecting drug users (IDUs) and the general community. For many countries, the costs far outweigh the benefits. The possible HIV-1 infection impact among IDUs is all important but a largely neglected consideration. The effectevness of supply reduction policy is unlikely to be increased significantly by allocation of greater resources, by more vigorous implementation. or by adoption of new technology. A range of alternative, credible options, including controlled availability, deserve consideration. Controlled availability is feasible and plausibly has greater benefits and fewer health, social, and economic costs than supply restriction. Innovative methods of providing currently illicit drugs to those who are determined to consume them deserve careful evaluation and comparison against current policies.

To decide whether current drug policy should be reviewed and possibly reformed requires that four basic questions be answered: 1) Is current policy working satisfactorily?; 2) If not, can it be modified to achieve satisfactory results; 3) If not, do feasible alternative options exist in comparison to present policy?; and 4) Are alternative options likely to be more effective than the present policy? Drug policy reform is desirable if the benefits of reform are to more significantly outweigh the costs than the benefits and costs arising from the present supply reduction policy. Policies always have to take local factors into account. A successful policy for Patagonia may be a disaster in Xanadu and vice versa.

It is difficult to resolve the impasse in the present drug policy debate without agreement on terms and objectives. Terms such as "legalization" and "decriminalization" are used widely but with a

bewildering variety of meanings. If legalization means the legal provision "of a drug of addiction to a person known to be an addict,"
then a form of legalization has been accepted for over two decades
in countries as diverse as the United States, Sweden, the United
Kingdom, and Australia where methadone maintenance programs
have become well accepted.

Much of the confusion in the vigorous debate over drug policy
results from a lack of clarity in the aims of the exercise. Should the
objective of national responses to illicit drugs be the reduction, or
elimination of drug use? If it is agreed that amelioration of the
harmful complications of drug use is the desired objective, then it
must be acknowledged that there are many ways by which this aim
can be achieved. The reduction or elimination of drug consumption is but one approach. Alternatively, the same objective of
reducing the sequelae of drug use could be achieved with unchang-
ing, or even increasing drug consumption if the drug use could be
rendered less hazardous. But if drug use is itself presumed to be evil
it follows logically that any consumption of specified drugs should
be reduced, or preferably, eliminated.

The question of whether drug consumption or drug-related harm
is the more appropriate target of government policy was clearly
answered in a recent major policy statement by the United States.

> We must come to terms with the drug problem in its essence: use
> itself. Worthy efforts to alleviate the symptoms of epidemic drug
> abuse – crime and disease, for example – must continue unabated.
> But a largely ad hoc attack on the holes in our dike can have
> only an indirect and minimal effect on the flood itself.[2]

It seems absurd, however, to consider the use of heroin or
cocaine as intrinsically evil. After all, several of the very drugs now
considered taboo had for many years been regarded as useful members of the pharmacopeia of a number of countries without any
question of their administration being considered a form of wicked-
ness. Harm resulting from drug use is the more appropriate target
of national and international drug policy, as was noted in an

authoritative statement of Australian policy. "[T]he aim is to minimize the harmful effects of drugs on Australian society."[3] Recognizing that the reduction of drug-related harm should be the intended objective of national drug policy and that decreasing drug consumption is but one possible means of achieving this end is the first step to a more rational approach to drug policy.

In order to decide whether reform of drug policy should even be considered, it is necessary to clarify first the intended benefits to be achieved and the specified costs to be avoided.[4] The adverse consequences of drug use can involve health, social and economic domains, and these must be considered separately for individuals and societies.

HEALTH COSTS ASSOCIATED WITH ILLICIT DRUGS

The pooled mortality rates for injecting drug users was estimated from 12 to be 9.6 deaths/1,000 persons-years, representing a relative risk compared to persons in the general population of similar age and sex of 17.1.[5] A far higher mortality rate, however, was recently reported of HIV-1 infected IDUs even before the onset of AIDS.[6] The injection of illicit drugs is, therefore, changing from what was once a slightly hazardous pastime to a high-risk behavior. In large parts of Europe, North America and Southeast Asia, this transition has already occurred.[7]

Overdose has always been a major cause of death associated with IDU, although distinguishing between accidental and suicide overdose is exceedingly difficult. Bacterial, viral, fungal, and parasitic infections continue to make an important contribution to morbidity and mortality in this population. In the era of AIDS, overdose still remains an important cause of death among IDUs and is possibly at least partly preventable because the concentration of is unknown. The uncertain concentration and microbiological chemical adulteration of street drugs are responsible for the majority of adverse health consequences of illicit drugs. The common practice of sharing injection equipment, which also contributes substantially to the spread of a number of blood-borne infections in this population, forms part of the subculture of IDUs. In recent years, encouraging progress was made in reducing the extent of sharing injection equipment in a number of countries.[8] Deficiencies in quality control of street drugs and unhygienic injection practices are exacerbated by the illegal status of street drugs and are not side-effects that can be reliably predicted from the pharmacology of the psychoactive ingredients. The health costs of drug use, however, are not restricted to IDUs. Several of the blood-bome infections such as hepatitis B or C are passed on from drug users to non-drug users. Non-drug using heterosexuals in most developing countries at present face the greatest risk of acquiring HIV-1 infection from sexual contact with an IDU.[9]

THE SOCIAL COST OF INJECTING DRUG USE

The social costs of drug use are both substantial and diverse. Although in many countries drug users span the socio-economic spectrum, the consumption of using illicit drugs seems to be both a consequence and cause of poverty. In addition, for many if not most consumers, the consequences of illicit drugs includes being at times ostracized from families, losing children, being unemployed, having unsatisfactory personal relationships, being an inadequate parent, and spending long periods in prison. But the social costs of drug use are also high for societies and such costs include the destruction of neighborhoods and rampant charity. Corruption of the criminal justice and political systems and infringement of civil liberties also seem to be common companions of supply reduction policies in many countries. None of these individual or community social costs can be attributed to the pharmacology of the drugs consumed. Rather, these costs stem from attempts to decrease drug use, or possibly to diminish drug-related harm by reducing drug use.

THE ECONOMIC COST OF INJECTING DRUG USE

The individual drug user pays an inflated price for intoxication from illicit compared to licit drugs. Most drug users, however, do not pay for the full cost of their drug use as this is largely passed on to non-drug users through property crime. It is difficult to estimate the full economic cost to society of illict drug use which covers law enforcement efforts directed to suppress cultivation, production, transport, sale, and consummation of specified substances; the expense of running courts and prisons; and insurance premiums and lost productivity. The cost of illicit drugs to the United States in 1983 was estimated to be $60 billion[10] representing about half the estimated cost of alcohol to the economy of the United States in the same year ($117 billion). It was conservatively estimated that in 1988 Australia spend A$258 million on law enforcement associated with illicit drugs.[11] This is equivalent to the annual cost in Austalia of either running a 1,200 bed-hospital incarceating 8,000 prisoners or keeping 100,000 patients in methadone maintenance treatment. Once again, these costs should not be regarded as the inevitable sequelae arising from the pharmacology of street drugs but rather as the costs incurred by law enforcement authorities intending to prevent the adverse consequences of illicit drug use.

THE BENEFITS OF ILLICIT DRUGS

It may seem perverse to consider even the possibility that illicit drugs could have benefits for some individuals or societies. But it is as important to assess the possible benefits of illicit drugs as it is to evaluate the effectiveness of attempts to diminish their supply. The global proceeds of the illicit drug industry now exceed $300 billion,[12] thus suggesting that there are major benefits for someone. Peasants growing opium poppies in areas where there are no roads, and doctors use opium as a traditional medicine to relieve pain, control diarrhea, and assuage hunger. For many families living in traditional growing areas, opium provides a few bright moments in a life of severe and unremitting hardship. For some, growing illicit drugs is a means of survival in a world of falling commodity prices and declining living standards. Whatever heroin may mean to communities and politicians in industrialized, and now some developing countries, for many farmers in the Golden Triangle and Golden Crescent, growing opium is a way of buying a kerosene lamp or bicycle or simply making ends meet. As stated in a recent U.S. report: "[P]easants have turned to cultivating the coca plan, because it is the most lucrative cash crop, offering in one season an income equivalent to a year's effort of growing traditional crops."[13] With an increasing number of third world countries trapped by mounting debt, cultivating illicit drugs is a way of making ends meet.

> [I]t cannot be denied that Colombians in general have benefited
> to some extent from the huge infusion of cash and capital
> brought about by the drug trade. It is believed, for example, that
> the Columbian Government was able to avoid rescheduling its
> foreign debt payments due to the positive economic effects of the
> drug boom.[14]

For the vast army of middle men, distributors, organizers, and the international underworld, there are rich pickings to be made from the transport and distribution of illicit drugs. This is not to commend or condone an illegal enterprise, but merely to note that there is a clear benefit to those willing to take the relatively small risks of heavy penalties which may result from successful detection and prosecution. The international terrorist organizations are also not unaware of the lucrative profits to be made from transporting a kilogram of heroin since its merchandise increases 1500 times. To the costs of attempting to diminish availability of illicit drugs should be added to the subsidy that this trade provides to a number of international terrorist organizations from the Shining Path (Sendoro Luminoso) of Peru to the Tamil Tigers in Sri Lanka. Illicit drugs also provide employment to an army of customs officers, police officers, lawyers and drug treatment staff. The fact that supply reduction policies generate substantial legal employment is a benefit that cannot be denied. It is also undisputable that many IDUs derive exquisite pleasure from the consumption of illicit drugs. Moreover, for residents of deprived inner city neighborhoods in some western countries, involvement in the distnbution of illic- it drugs provides one of the few available albeit illusory escape routes from a lifetime of squalor, unemployment, and poverty.

THE EFFECTIVENESS OF SUPPLY REDUCTION POLICIES

Although one of the major objectives of attempts to restrict the supply of illicit drugs is the reduction of availability, it is difficult to find convincing evidence of a sustained decrease in the supply of psychoactive substances following the application of this policy. The vagaries of weather seem more likely than law enforcement efforts to decrease the global availability of drugs. A recent official U.S. report concluded that "global production of opium increased each year during the last decade and more than doubled between 1986 and 1990."[15] Global coca production increased 25% between 1989 and 1990.[16] The report continued by stating that "although precise info is difficult to obtain, it seems clear that worldwide abuse of drugs is increasing. A number of countries reported or were estimated to have more drug abuse problems than in previous years."[17] It is not difficult to understand why supply reduction pol- icy has been so unsuccessful. A study of the economics of drug mar- kets and their interaction with law enforcement authorities observed that "[t]he 'success' of law enforcement in maintaining high prices is also its Achilles heel, creating extraordinary opportu- nities for extraordinary profits thereby attracting entrepreneurs whom the law seeks to discourage by enforcement of the very law(s) which created profitable markets and attracted entrepre- neurs in the first place."[18]

If evidence of the effectiveness of supply reduction policy in decreasing drug availability or drug-related problems is lacking, can there be any confidence that intensification or some other modification would be more successful? A recent study funded by the U.S. Department of Defense estimated the impact of increasing the effectiveness of interdiction of cocaine from 20% to 50% and determined that this would result in only a 4% increase in cocaine prices.[19] An earlier comprehensive review of strategies for controlling adolescent drug use in the United States concluded that "further increases in law enforcement is not likely to substantially reduce drug use"[20] and "more intense law enforcement is not likely to substantially affect either the availability or the retail price of drugs in this country."[21] It is difficult to believe that the lack of evidence of the effectiveness of supply reduction policy reflects either insufficient allocation of resources, a reluctance to adopt stern measures, or patience in the effect of policies. Has the time not come to conclude that supply on policies neither restrict significantly the availability of drugs nor decrease the incidence of drug-related problems? Can there be any confidence that intensification of application or other modification of these policies will be more effective? As George Schultz, former U.S. Secretary of State concluded, "the conceptual base of the current program is flawed and the program is not likely to work ... We need at least to consider and examine forms of controlled legalization of drugs."[22]

ALTERNATIVES TO SUPPLY REDUCTION POLICY

Is there an alternative to supply reduction policy? The choice for policy-makers is more extensive than selecting between existing policy and legalization. A range of options is available.[23] Under total prohibition, the cultivation, production, use, possession, and sale of drugs are all prohibited and regarded as a criminal offense.[23] In the second option of modified total prohibition which is also referred to as "decriminalization," personal use session, and cultivation for personal use are defined, as illegal but only attract nominal fines.[25] Supply is still regarded as a criminal offense, but the minimum quantity linked to a penalty can be varied. A third policy option is partial prohibition where personal use and cultivation are not considered an offense.[26]   Public use, commercial cultivation and sale, however, remain illegal and subject to a set of variable fines. A fourth option is a user license system whereby some form of controlled use is permitted following the issuance of a license or registration.[27] A fifth option is free availability where there are minimal or no restrictions on availability.[28] These options originate from a Canadian Royal Commision on cannabis,[29] but they apply equally well to other illicit drugs, or for that matter, to legal drugs.

Most western countries in the nineteenth century permitted the use of currently illicit substances with relatively few regulations. In some countries opium and later cocaine-containing compounds could be obtained from grocery stores and later from retail pharmacies. The foundation of the present system of supply reduction began with an International Conference in Hague in 1912.[30] This system has progressively intensified in recent decades by a number of international treaties and a proliferation of international regulatory authorities. There is little likelihood of returning to the nineteenth century laissez-faire system for psychoactive substances even though this was associated with relatively stable levels of consumption and apparently few opium or cocaine-related problems.[31] Speculation about a possible return to free availability is unhelpful as it is exceedingly unlikely that any western country in foreseeable future could ever gather sufficient political support to countenance such a move or be able to extricate itself from relevant international treaty obligations. The development of rapid transport of goods between potential producer and consumer countries, ready availability of multiple use cheap injection equipment and substantial third world debt may be some of the factors which prevent a return to the halcyon policies of yesteryear. But the association between the laissez-faire policies of western countries in the nineteenth century with relatively few observed problems contrasts starkly with the contemporary situation in which a plethora of response-related sequelae are all too evident and problems which are directly consequent on the pharmacology of illicit substances are remarkable for their comparative rarity.

The likelihood of success of a prohibition policy depends on the demand for the psychoactive substance, the scope for illicit cultivation, production or concealed transport, and the availability of possible substitutes with similar properties. Prohibition can be a successful policy, as in the case of Mandrax (methaqualone-melsedin), where demand was modest, domestic productions were difficult, and other psychoactive substances were readily available.

An alternative option to current policy which must be seriously considered is the controlled availability of current illicit substances. Such a system has been implemented m the United Kingdom to a greater or lesser extent since the 1926 Rolleston Royal Commission advised that prescribing opium for addicts was reasonable if the patient could not be withdrawn without serious withdrawal symptoms; if the patient was undergoing a gradual withdrawal; or if the patient needed the drug to lead a useful and normal life.[31] A similar approach was adopted in the United States when intravenous morphine was supplied to registered drug addicts from a number of centers across the country during the 1920s.[31] Morphine maintenance in the United States was regarded as a generally reputable operation, but the program came to an abrupt end because it was seen to be irreconcilable with the prevailing spirit of the prohibition of alcohol.[34]

In Britain, intravenous heroin, cocaine, and amphetamines have all at times been legally prescribed since the Rolleston Royal Commission. The prescribing of oral methadone has become far more popular since the 1960s and prescribing of intravenous heroin, cocaine, and amphetamines in now uncommon. The only publishable study comparing the effectiveness of oral methadone and intravenous heroin produced equivocal results.[35] The Drug Dependency Clinic in Widnes, an outer suburb of Liverpool, briefly reported their innovative approach.[36] Following a clinical assessment, selected patients are provided with either oral methadone or heroin, cocaine or amphetamines in intravenous or smokable form. Unintended negative consequences have not been reported. As no formal external evaluation is yet available, it is not possible to say whether this clinic has been more successful in reducing the complications of street drug use than have other approaches. It is undeniable, however, that this policy is operationally feasible. It is possible to select patients who are suitable for this kind of treatment, chose to prescribe certain drugs and not others, and decide on the dose to be prescribed. Such innovative approaches need to be carefully and independently evaluated. It can be concluded confidently from the historical and contemporary experience with controlled availability in the United States[37] and United Kingdom[38] that this is a feasible alternative. Comparing the costs and benefits of controlled availability with supply reduction policy, however, requires more information than is available presently.

The spread of HIV-1 infection now presents the most serious complication of drug injecting both for IDUs and non-drug users alike was noted in a Scottish report soon after an epidemic of HIV was detected in Edinburgh that "the gravity of the problem is such that on balance the containment of the spread of the virus is a higher priority in management than the prevention of drug misuse."[39] Drug policy, therefore, also needs to be considered from the perspective of the known or likely impact of HIV-1 transmission.[40] In the absence of any panacea, least worst solutions are the appropriate goal of the policy maker.

PLAUSIBILITY OF CONTROLLED AVAILABILITY

By supplying pharmacological preparations of currently illicit drugs in known concentrations together with sterile injection equipment, it is reasonable to assume that the number of deaths from accidental overdose, and microbiological and chemical contamination will be reduced substantially. As these are currently the major causes of heroin-related, or more correctly prohibition-related, heath problems, a reduction in morbidity and mortality among IDUs is plausible. By supplying ancillary vocational and counseling services to a larger proportion of drug users attracted into treatment by a greater diversity of options, it is likely that improved rehabilitation will also be achieved. Achieving a greater participation rate of illicit drug users in treatment is likely to lessen the social cost of drug use for individual drug users well as for the broader community. If the cost of running a vastly expanded treatment service responsible for dispensing intravenous heroin, cocaine, and amphetamines similar to that of oral methadone programs, the expenditure, required is likely to be far less than that currently allocated to law enforcement responses to street drugs because drug treatment is far cheaper than incarceration.

Law enforcement will always have a critical role to play in response to currently illicit drugs just as it forms an important component to the control of legal drugs. Although there is insufficient evidence at present, and such evidence will probably never become available to compare directly the costs and benefits of current policies with controlled availability of illicit drugs with corresponding less emphasis on supply reduction would almost certainly result in a decrease in crime, less corruption, and fewer infringements upon civil liberties. An essentially health and welfare response would replace the current emphasis on law enforcement.

Unintended negative consequences of new policies would need to be anticipated and minimized. The difficulties of introducing controlled availability in Britain in the sixties and seventies should give pause for thought.[41] Were these difficulties the inevitable result of controlled availability, or were they peculiar to the system adopted? The lack of reports of similar difficulties in the sizeable morphine maintenance program implemented in the United States[42] suggests that these problems are not inevitable companions to controlled availability. A widespread system of controlled availability will almost certainly put more strain on the reputability of medical practice. Clearer guidelines and improved surveillance of doctors would probably need to be introduced. The financial savings resulting from the treatment of illicit drugs largely as a health and welfare, rather than as a law enforcement matter are likely to be substantial.

THE EFFECT OF CHANGING POLICY ON THE NUMBER OF DRUG USERS

One of the most prominent and persistent fears about any change in policy is the possibility that an increase in the numbers of persons using currently illicit drugs would follow reform. Unfortunately, we can only speculate as to the effect of changing policies on the number of drug users in a community. The experience of liberalizing policies on cannabis in a few states of the United States provides some guidance. No increase in marijuana use was attributed to decriminalization but costs of law enforcement and prosecution fell.[43] The number of person consuming drugs should at any rate be less of a concern than the incidence and severity of drug-related harm.[44]

If a system of controlled availability resulted in an increase in the number of drug-users and we have no reason to suppose that this would be the case, but the incidence and severity of drug-related ham decreased because drug use became safer, this should be regarded as a positive outcome. And if the number of drug users remained unchanged, but drug-related harm decreased because drug use had become safer, would this not be a consummation devoutly to be wished?

Supply reduction drug policies are supposed to suppress drug use by increasing the retail cost of illicit drugs through maintaining a high risk of arrest, prosecution, and punishment. This approach is also purported to deter drug use by raising the health and social costs of illicit drug consumption for consumers although again a considerable proportion of these penalties are passed on to the general community.

As a consequence of a supply reduction approach to illicit drugs a pyramidal distribution system is established with user-dealers required to recruit new consumers to offset the high use of drop. This type of distribution is an extremely efficient retailing system for merchandise where a monopoly of supply exits. It is difficult to imagine a more efficient system for recruiting drug users into a wholesale and retail illicit drugs distribution network than a supply-restriction drug policy which inadvertently ensures that the harm consequent on drug consumption for drug users and the general community alike is maximized. One of the extraordinary features of the current drug policy debate is the failure to acknowledge the importance of market forces at a time when historical events taking place across the world serve to emphasize that they cannot be ignored.

CONCLUSION

The increasing costs and limited effectiveness of present attempts to control the supply of drugs ultimately will force many countries to consider credible options. A system of controlled availability appears to be a feasible alternative worthy of consideration and careful evaluation.

Fundamentally, the choice for many countries lies between the present policy of supply restriction, which leads to criminals selling contaminated drugs of unknown concentration indiscriminately to any person who can meet the purchase price, and a system of controlled availability involving the dealing of sterile drugs of known concentration to selected drug users who could be supervised and offered other forms of assistance. A system of controlled availability would not eliminate all of the many unhappy consequences of illicit drugs. It would not, for example represent a satisfactory answer to recreational drug use. On present evidence, however, it can be concluded confidently that taking up arms against a sea of drugs does not by opposing them end them.

DEBATE QUESTIONS:

What are the 'four basic questions' the author feels need to be answered 'to decide whether current drug policy should be reviewed and possibly reformed'? Do these four basic questions seem right to you? What might be other questions?

This author clearly feels that 'harm resulting from drug use is the more appropriate target of national and international policy.' Can there still be a place for aiming to reduce consumption?

Which one of the 'range of options' that do not involve reducing supply seems most viable to you? Does the author seem to favor one approach instead of others? If he does, do you agree?

NOTES

[1] Journal of Contemporary Health Law and Policy, 1993; 9:323.
[2] Office of National Drug Policy, Executive Office of the President, National Drug Control Strategy 8 (1989).
[3] Department of Health, National Campaign Against Drug Abuse 2 (1985).
[4] See Ethan A. Nadelman, Drug Prohibition in the United States: Costs, Consequences, and Alternatives 245 Science 939-47 (1989) ("Drug legalization policies that are wisely implemented can minimize the risks of legalization, dramatically reduce the costs of current policies, and directly address the problems of drug abuse.")
[5] See C.D.J. Homan et al., Commonwealth Dep't of Community Servs. & Health, The Quanitification of Drug Caused Morbidity and Mortality in Australia (1990).
[6] Rand L. Stoneburner et al. A Larger Spectrum of Severe HIV-1 Related Disease in Injeting Drug Users in New York City 242 Science 916, 918-19 (1988).
[7] Alex Wodak & A. Moss, HIV-1 Infection and Intravenous Drug Users: From Epidemiology to Public Heath, 4 AIDS 105-109 (1990)
[8] R.P. Brettle, HIV and Harm Reduction for Injection Drug Users, 5 AIDS 125-136 (1990).
[9] Don C. Jerlais et al. HIV Infection and Intravenous Drug Use: Critical Issues in Transmission Dynamics, Infection Outcomes and Prevention, 10 Rev. Infectious Diseases 151-53 (1988). In New York City, 87% of the cases of heterosexual transmission have occurred from an IV drug user to a sexual partner who does not inject drugs. Id. at 152.

[10] *See generally* Research Triangle Institute, Alcohol, Drug Abuse & Mental Health Admin., U.S. Dep't of Health, Economic Costs to Society of Alcohol and Drug Abuse and Mental Illness (1986).

[11] D.J. Collins & H.M. Lapsley, National Campaign Against Drug Abuse Estimating the Economic Costs of Drug Abuse in Australia 86 (1991).

[12] Bureau of International Narcotic Matter, U.S. Dep't of State, International Narcotics Control Strategy Report 48 (1990) [hereinafter Narcotic Matter]

[13] Office of Atty. Gen., U.S. Dep't of Justice, Drug Trafficking: A Report to the President of the United States 19 (1989)

[14] *Id.* at 20

[15] Narcotic Matter, at 13

[16] *Id.*

[17] *Id.*

[18] Steven Wisotsky, *Breaking the Impasse in the War on Drugs* 32 (1986).

[19] *See generally* Peter Reuter et al., *Sealing the Borders: the Effects of Increased Military Participation in Drug Interdiction* (1988).

[20] J. Michael Polich et al, *Strategies for Controlling Adolescent Drug Use* 155 (1984).

[21] *Id.* at 157.

[22] *Schulz on Drug Legilation*, Wall Et. J., Oct. 27, 1991, at A16.

[23] *See* Greg Chesher & Alex Wodak, *Evolving a New Policy for Illicit Drugs*, 20 J. Drug Issues 555-61 (1990) (stating that these alternative policies offer greater individual and societal benefits and fewer negative consequences). The options include: decriminalization; a selective moratorium on the application of drug laws as they apply to the drug users; availability on prescription by a medical practitioner; a legal market with controls similar to those presently exercised on alcohol and tobacco; regulated availability. *Id.* at 556-59

[24] *Id.* at 556

[25] *Id.*

[26] *Id.* at 557

[27] Id. at 558

[28] *Id.* at 559-60

[29] Gerald Le Dain et al. Gov't of Canada, Report of the Commission of Inquiry into the Non-Medical Use of Drugs 10 (1972) (discussing the treatment of opiate dependents) [hereinafter Le Dain Commission]

[30] David F.D. Musto, *The American Disease: Origins of Narcotic Control* 49-52 (1973); K. Bruun et al., *The Gentleman's Club: International Control of Drugs and Alcohol* 1 (1975).

[31] *See* Virginia Berridge & Griffith Edwards, *Opium and the People: Opium Use in Nineteenth Century England* (1981).

[32] Rolleston Committee, Ministry of Health, Report of Departmental Committee on Morphine and Heroine Addiction 19 (1926).

[33] Musto, at 49-52

[34] Le Dain Commission, at 10.

[35] *See generally* Richard L. Hartnol et al., *Evaluation of Heroin Maintenance in Controlled Trial*, 37 Archives Gen. Psychiatry 877-84 (1980). This study tested IDU's response to a maintenance program when treated with injectable heroin

or oral methadone. *Id.* at 877.

[36] J.A. Marks, *The North Wind and the Sun*, 21 Proceedings Royal Coll. Physicians Edinburgh 319-27 (1991).

[37] Musto, at 49-52

[38] Marks, at 319

[39] *See generally* Scottish Home & Health Dep't, *HIV Infection in Scotland: Report of the Scottish Committee on HIV Infection and Intravenous Drug Misuse* (1986).

[40] Alex Wodak, *The Connection Between HIV Infection in Injecting Drug Users and Drug Policy*, 1 Int'l J. Drug Pol'y 22-23 (1990).

[41] Gerry A. Stimson & Edna Oppenheimer, *Heroin Addiction: Treatment and Control in Britain* 49 (1982).

[42] Musto, at 49-52

[43] Eric W. Single, *The Impact of Marijuana Decriminalization: An Update*, 1989 J. Pub. Health Pol'y 457, 462 (1989).

[44] *Id.* at 462-63

Part 3
Human Rights aspects

Whereas the relevant policy question is usually "Can we do this?" questions concerning human rights are often more rightly framed as "Should we do this?". The following four articles address the important intersection where drug use, disease, and human rights meet. "When, if ever, does personal privacy trump public concerns?" "Are people with HIV/AIDS unfairly discriminated against?" These are the types of questions these articles tackle. You may find it helpful to refer to Part 4 when reading through these articles, as Part 4 includes many relevant international documents concerning human rights, disease, and drug use. Again, at the end of each article, you will find debate/discussion questions to spur your thinking.

Impact of Legal and Public Policy Measures to Control Drug Use on Human Rights

Norbert Gilmore, Professor McGill University Centre for Medicine, Ethics and Law

Human rights are usually defined as the basic unalienable rights of individuals that are protected by several international conventions and agreements, including the Universal Declaration on Human Rights (see Human Rights Treaties and Guidelines), International Covenant on Civil and Political Rights, International Covenant on Economic, Social and Cultural Rights (see Human Rights Treaties and Guidelines). However, of all the rights in the human rights catalogue, the right to privacy is the most difficult to define. This right is extremely important, thus it is protected by national and international legislation, and one can claim that this right is being violated with the prosecution of drug users for their consumption behavior. Some defined privacy as the desire of people to choose freely when and under what circumstances, as well as to what extent they will expose themselves to others. Some would define "privacy" as an individual claim to limit access by others to some aspect of her personal life. The term is very vague and embraces the freedom of decision-making about one's bodily integrity without interference, and the right not to be viewed and photographed as well as "informational privacy" as an individual's right to control the disclosure of personal health information.

There is a strong belief among human rights advocates around the world that the privacy- based approach towards drug use can be beneficial both to drug users and the health care system.

The analysis of legal and public policy responses to drug use suggests several conclusions, (1) legal and policy responses are dynamic and evolving; (2) there is increasing appreciation for the salience of harm-reducing, public health approaches to these responses; (3) there is a scarcity of discourse about drug use and human rights and an urgent need for analysis of the intersection of drug use and human rights; (4) human rights concepts and principles can provide useful insights into legal and policy responses to drug use; and (5) there are at least four situations in which the present legal and public policy responses to drug use have impact on the human rights of drug users.

The first situation concerns the value of privacy in relation to drug use and infringement on privacy by government efforts to control drug use.[1] The threshold issue about whether or not drug use can be considered a "private" activity and, if so, under what circumstances and what limitations might there be on government intervention aimed at controlling drug use?

The second situation relates to reduced respect for the human rights of drug users. Unlike nonusers, many drug users are marginalized, often impoverished, and are often stigmatized, scapegoated, and discriminated against prior to using drugs, and they are made even more so by their drug use. It is not uncommon that people in such situations will exclude themselves from society, fail to seek respect for their rights, and forgo exercising them, even when opportunities to exercise their rights are available. The adverse influences to which they are prey become a self-fulfilling prophecy.[2]

The third situation relates to the impairment of the health and autonomy of drug users, particularly their mental health. This concern poses three questions. First, what protection do drug users need as a result of these impairments?[3] Second, can drug users be considered disabled, and therefore eligible for the same protection afforded other disabled persons?[4] Finally, under what conditions could drug use be considered a disabling condition?[5]

The fourth situation concerns discrimination against drug users and violations of their human rights based on their use of drugs. While both human rights violations and discrimination against drug users appear to be common, there is a scarcity of empirical data documenting these abuses. Consequently, there is a need to identify and characterize situations in which such abuses can or are likely to occur.[6]

A. DRUG USE AS A PRIVATE BEHAVIOR

Drug use is a very widespread behavior. It can occur openly as with tobacco and alcohol use, furtively as with cannabis, LSD, or XTC use, or clandestinely as with amphetamine, cocaine, and heroin. Each of these activities is an individual behavior that has a variable impact on the user and others. In this regard, drug use is similar to many other private behaviors. The following section argues that drug use can be considered a private behavior like many other daily activities. In doing so, it recognizes that:

> There are broader and narrower conceptions of privacy. On the narrower range of conceptions, privacy relates exclusively to information of a personal sort about an individual and describes the extent to which others have access to this information. A broader conception extends beyond the informational domain and encompasses anonymity and restricted physical access .... Embracing some aspects of autonomy within the definition of privacy, it has been defined as control over the intimacies of personal identity. At the broadest end of the spectrum, privacy is thought to be the measure of the extent an individual is afforded the social and legal space to develop the emotional, cognitive, spiritual, and moral powers of an autonomous agent. An advocate of one of the narrower conceptions can agree about the value of autonomous development but think that privacy as properly defined makes an important but limited contribution to its achievement.

Privacy is important as a means of respecting or even socially constructing moral personality, compromising qualities like independent judgement, creativity, self-knowledge, and self-respect. It is important because of the way control over one's thoughts and body enables one to develop trust for, or love and friendship with, one another and more generally modulate relationships with others. It is important too for the political dimensions of a society that respects individual privacy, finding privacy instrumental in protecting rights of association, individual freedom, and limitations on governmental control over thoughts and actions. Finally, it has been argued that privacy is important as a means of protecting people from overreaching social (as opposed to legal) pressures and sanctions and is thus critical if people are to enjoy a measure of social freedom.[7]

The classification of drug use as a private behavior depends upon showing that it is an autonomous activity and that it does not differ substantially from other private activities. This necessitates first distinguishing between innocuous, voluntary drug use and that which is compulsive and harmful. Second, the similarities between drug use and other private activities must be determined. This requires an analysis of the benefits, risks, and harms associated with drug use and other activities.

1. VOLUNTARY, "INOCUOUS" DRUG USE

Many activities exist that are considered private and involve individuals acting autonomously. Society seldom interferes with such activities.[8] Generally, the activities in which autonomous individuals[9] are free to use their own bodies for their own purposes include those where engaging in the activity does not cause excessive harm to themselves or others.[10] This includes tolerating and sometimes encouraging a wide variety of sports and leisure activities (e.g., adventuring, drinking coffee and alcohol, smoking tobacco, the use of computer and video games, playing bingo, and casino and race-track gambling), despite the occurrence of tragedies, injuries, or other avoidable harms which can sometimes result from these activities. Society, by not prohibiting these activities, implicitly views the benefits of such activities as outweighing the harms that may occur from them.[11] On the other hand, drug use, like smoking and the immoderate use of alcohol, is generally condemned and punished by governments.[12] Nonetheless, large numbers of people use drugs illicitly, and most of them do so without causing serious harm to themselves, other than breaking the law regarding their use. Moreover, apart from the indirect harms to society related to the interdiction of drugs, society is seldom harmed by this activity.

Despite a widespread exception that drug use is dangerous and harmful, there is ample data supporting a conclusion that, on the basis of all types of drug users, most drug use is transient, noncompulsive, and innocuous.[13] For example, a recent study of individuals with private health insurance in New York estimated that one percent of the total insurance subscriber population studied were steadily employed, opiate-using individuals.[14] According to the U.S. Department of Labor, 77 percent of "serious cocaine users" are regularly employed. In surveys of students in the United States, 3.1% reported that they had used cocaine and 5.6% had used LSD during 1992.[15] In Canada, almost five percent of men and slightly less than two percent of women between the ages of twenty-five and thirty-four reported that they had used cocaine during 1989 and approximately four percent of adults reported using LSD, methamphetamine ("speed"), or heroin at least once.[16] Even more alarming, however, was that 1.3% of Canadians reported that they had injected themselves with drugs using needles shared with someone else.[17] Given such findings, it is not unreasonable to conclude that most drug use is undertaken voluntarily. Nevertheless, such activity, even if voluntary, may not always be undertaken harmlessly or under conditions of minimum risk. However, drugs can be used in a manner that is not seriously harmful to users or to others. This poses the question whether or not government intrusion into this behavior is justifiable and, if so, under what conditions might it be justifiable? This has obvious implications regarding the opportunities of drug users to exercise their rights *viz a viz* government intervention to control this behavior.

Drug use can be viewed as a particular example of a more generalized principle; namely, that despite the risks, people use their bodies in a variety of ways for their own private intimate, and voluntary purposes, including pleasure.[18] Many of these activities are prevalent and popular. Examples include alpine skiing, whitewater rafting, bungee-jumping, sunbathing, racetrack betting, and social drinking. Some of these activities can be risky and, indeed, some people engage in them because they are both exhilarating and dangerous. Nevertheless, governments do not prohibit these activities and rarely interfere with them, other than to regulate them in order to reduce or prevent the risks harms they present. This leads to the question of whether or not voluntary, innocuous drug use can be considered distinct from such activities with regard to their benefits, risks, and harms. If drug use differs substantively from these other activities, dissimilar treatment is justified. On the other hand, if drug use is not dissimiliar, only those aspects of drug use differing from these other activities warrant different treatment. Because it is difficult to identify substantive differences in benefits, risks, and harms between voluntary, innocuous drug use and other comparable private activities, it would not be unreasonable to conclude that voluntary, innocuous drug use is a private, albeit risky, and sometimes, harmful behavior.

One consequence of a *prima facie* presumption that drug use is a private activitiy is that legal and public policy responses to drug use cannot be treated differently from responses to other private behavior.[19] In other words, government responses to drug use have to be consistent with those of other comparable behaviors. Here, proportionality is concerened with "whether the legislative response to illicit drug behaviour is appropriate relative to the state response to other particularly harmful behaviors .... Proportionality, like the efficient allocation of limited enforcement resources, includes comparison with other risk-producing conduct and the subsequent comparison of drug-related behaviours relative to one another."[20] On the other hand, equality demands that like cases be treated alike or "that the legal definitions of offences correspond to meaningful categories of human behaviour."[21] This has, at least, four important human rights implications.

First, considering drug use to be a private behavior would seriously question the prohibition of voluntary and innocuous (in contrast to compulsive or harmful) drug use. This, however, does not imply that people have a "right" to use drugs. As one commentator has noted:

> One reason to deny that adults have a moral right to use recreational drugs is that the principle of autonomy does not apply to protect any recreational activity. According to this school of thought, no one has a right to play baseball, ski, or participate in any nonprofessional sport. Persons are morally permitted to engage in recreational persuits only as long as consequentialist considerations allow them to do so. But as soon as a net balance of disutility is caused by a given recreational activity, the state would have the authority to prohibit it without infringing moral rights.[22]

It also does not imply that governments cannot prohibit or limit the use of a drug when it would have a serious and unavoidable net harm for the user or for others. It would mean, however, that prohibiting or limiting the use of a drug would be the least restrictive and intrusive intervention available to prevent the risks and harms of drug use. For example, in ruling on a claim that marijuana use at home is constitutionally protected by a right to privacy, the Alaska Supreme Court held that:

> [T]he authority of the state to exert control over the individual extends only to activities of the individual as it relates to matters of public health or safety, or to provide for the general welfare. We believe this tenet to be basic to a free society. The state cannot impose its own notions of morality, propriety, or fashion on individuals when the public has no legitimate interest in the affairs of those individuals.[23]

The standard applicable to state intervention aimed at preventing or reducing the risks and harms from drug use would, presumably, not differ from that which applies to state intervention into other private behavior. This would mean that an intervention to prohibit or limit drug use is (1) the least intrusive and least restrictive measure reasonably available; (2) proportional to the benefits, risks, and harms involved; and (3) not disproportionate to interventions for other comparable private behaviors. Because private behaviors, including drug use, can be compared to those of other behaviors insofar as their benefits, risks, and harms are similar, and differ only insofar as their benefits, risks, and harms differ. Unfortunately, responses to drug use rarely recognize such a standard. This is illustrated by responses to the use of tobacco, alcohol, and many narcotics, as well as to prohibited drugs such as cannabis, methadone, and heroin. The harms from the chronic use of tobacco and alcohol, on both a population basis and individually, exceeded the harms of most, if not all, prohibited drugs, as well as the harms associated with many private activities. Despite this, tobacco and alcohol use are not prohibited in most societies except for their sale to and consumption by minors, while the use of many less harmful drugs is banned. Further, activities such as scuba diving, bungee jumping, and skydiving are rarely prohibited.

Second, considering drug use to be a private behavior would shift the emphasis of government intervention from primarily controlling the supply and use of drugs to that of preventing or reducing the risks and harms resulting from drug use. This would be consistent with other "positive content" human rights obligations of governments, such as preventing and protecting from disease. Examples of such interventions include educating drug users about the risks and harms of drug use, providing drug users with opportunities to avoid using drugs or to use them in a harmless manner, and helping to make available and accessible the care and treatment that drug users who use drugs in a harmful manner may need. Subject to the availability of resources, these interventions would likely entail counseling, providing clean injection equipment, and treatment such as methadone maintenance.

Third, viewing drug use as a private behavior would avoid or reduce situations in which rights would be jeopardized or infringed. This would reduce activities aimed at the detection of individuals possessing or using drugs, such as drug testing, searches, and seizures.

Fourth, considering drug use to be a private behavior would help decrease the stigmatization and scapegoating of drug users. This, in turn, would help ensure that the benefits, risks, and harms associated with the use of drugs would be more accurately assessed. Implicit in such an assessment is the importance of preventing and reducing risks and harms. It would also counterbalance the widely held belief that drug use is a public menace or danger. When drug users are perceived to be immoral, weak, and prey to inescapably dangerous drugs, the public perceives itself as needing to be protected from drugs and, all too often, from those who use them, In such a setting, prohibition, abstinence, and mandatory treatment are perceived as being necessary. It is believed that drug users need to be controlled, isolated, or confined, either by self-isolation or social exclusion, or by imprisonment. Such beliefs can easily lead to the passage and persistence of laws that reinforce these views.

Considering drug use to be a private activity is not a novel idea. Although they recognize the risks and harms involved, so governments already consider the use of some drugs to be a private matter. Perhaps the most prominent example of such a response is the response of governments to tobacco and alcohol use. Almost every community forcefully prohibits individuals from driving under the influence of alcohol, yet drinking alcohol is not permitted. At the same time, governments educate people about the risks and harms from drinking alcohol, label bottles containing alcohol with health promoting messages, and encourage treatment when alcohol use is compulsive. This response to alcohol use illustrates the powerful impact of stigmatization. Alcohol abuse is strongly stigmatized, yet in most cultures its moderate use is unstigmatized (as alcohol advertising demonstrates). In contrast, the illicit use of most prohibited drugs is despised and severely penalized – even when these drugs are used with great moderation and at minimal risk to the user and others.

That some drug users may become seriously dependent upon drugs would not appear to negate a *prima facie* presumption that drug use is a private behavior, because while dependence is s risk, it is not an unavoidable or inescapably harmful consequence of drug use. Many drug users can and do use drugs, often over long periods of time, without necessarily becoming harmfully dependent on them. Serious compulsive drug use is a harm similar to the harms that can occur from other private, voluntary activities, which may be strictly regulated but not prohibited.

Viewing drug use to be a private behavior would help erode the false dichotomy by which alcohol and tobacco use are perceived to differ from the use of other drugs. All drugs would be viewed as potentially harmful, but able to be used in ways that can avoid or minimize these harms. It would also help to reduce stereotyping of drug use as inherently "evil," morally offensive, and unavoidably harmful, thereby helping to reduce stigmatization, scapegoating, and discrimination against drug users and the communities to which they belong. Society would then view those who use drugs in a harmful manner as individuals needing help, rather than as individuals deserving punishment for engaging in a clandestine, criminal behavior. It would also provide a more coherent and rational perspective on the distinction between the personal use of drugs and drug trafficking. Finally, it would distinguish risks and harms from current legal and public policy responses aimed at controlling drug use from those related to drug use itself.

2. COMPULSIVE AND LIKELY HARMFUL DRUG USE

This autonomy-emphasizing approach to drug use must be undertaken with caution because there is no clear demarcation between when drug use is voluntary and innocuous and when it is compulsive and likely to be harmful. The autonomy of drug users and the voluntariness of their drug use can be eroded when their drug use is persistent and becomes compulsive.[24] Most people would probably agree that sometimes state intervention aimed at preventing or minimizing this risk and its harms is needed, justifiable, and desirable, but there seems to be little agreement about what should be the limits on such interventions. Views of what can and should be done to control the risks and harms of drug use are often not balanced, but often usually extreme and polarized. On the one hand, proponents of prohibition claim that an absolute ban on drug use is necessary and justifiable in view of the risks and harms brought about by drug use. They support these views, seemingly without regard to the costs and other harms which can result from prohibition, including the creation of a false dichotomy between licit and illicit drug use rather than harmless and harmful drug use. On the other hand, there are those who would restrict state intervention to those that regulate the availability of and accessibility to drugs only when drugs are likely to be used in a harmful manner. There are numerous examples of such nonprohibitionary intrusions into private life, including age restrictions, licensing, limiting the sale and consumption of alcohol to certain hours, banning the smoking of tobacco at public venues, breathalyzer testing, and severe penalties for driving or working when under the influence of drugs. There are particular scenarios that illustrate responses that minimize interference with the human rights of drug users when intervention is deemed necessary.

First, there is the situation in which drug use can be innocuous for the user, but harmful to others. For example, when a pregnant woman uses drugs, including tobacco and alcohol, it can be relatively innocuous for her yet dangerous to her fetus.[25] The least intrusive and restrictive response to such a situation would be to persuade pregnant women to stop using drugs when they are pregnant. The most intrusive-restrictive response would be to coerce pregnant women to voluntarily forgo using drugs when pregnant. The former approach, which involves education, counseling, outreach, and support, avoids the counter-productive risk of driving pregnant users underground and discouraging them from seeking health care which they and their fetus need. Only when the less intrusive-restrictive approaches are unsuccessful, should more restrictive approaches be employed to protect the fetus.[26] Although neither response is incompatible with prohibiting pregnant women from using drugs, the former, noncoercive response views pregnant drug users as needing help to strengthen or reinforce their autonomy to stop using drugs and that the use of coercion is a "last resort" intervention.

Second, there are situations where the autonomy of the drug user may be impaired or undeveloped such as when children use drugs. The early use of drugs has been associated with subsequent, harmful drug use. Thus, users who develop dependence on or compulsive use of drugs at a younger age are more prone to develop these problems, while those who initiate drug use at a later age are less likely to have the same problem.[27] The least intrusive and least restrictive response to this situation would be "positive content" interventions. This type of intervention can increase children's awareness of drugs risks and harms, enhance their self-esteem and ability to resist using drugs, and teach them skills to abstain from drug use or to use them is a safe manner. This may involve, for example, mandatory school education about drug use, advice, accurate information, counseling, support, care, and the promotion of peer-regulation. Further treatment may be necessary to protect children who otherwise may be unable to avoid drug use.[28] At the same time, the role of parents and guardians in determining what should be done to their children must be recognized. Even if parents or guardians refuse such interventions, these interventions are likely to remain justifiable, but the scope of the resulting intrusion would be increased.

Third, situations exist in which individuals are placed at risk of serious harm by drug users. In such situations, warning the imperiled individuals of their risk may be necessary despite the intrusion into their private life. This scenario is analogous to notifying the sexual partners of individuals with a sexually transmissable disease or people exposed to someone with a communicable disease such as tuberculosis.[29] For example, it may be appropriate to warn an employer about a heavy equipment operator if that employee's drug use is likely to endanger others when using drugs. Similarly, the friends or family of a drug user may need to be informed if the drug user were prone to abusive behavior or a mental health disorder. This would be necessary if the disorder is triggered or aggravated by using drugs and the drug user refuses to heed advice about this risk.

Fourth, there are situations in which the mandatory treatment of drug users may be necessary and justifiable in order to avoid or reduce the risk of harm to others. Generally, these situations involve compulsive drug use. However, situations may exist where mandatory treatment of noncompulsive drug use would be the only effective means to protect others from serious harm. For the most part, these situations arise when a drug user repeatedly places others at risk of serious harm from physical sexual abuse, violence, or trauma that would be unlikely or nonexistent in the absence of drug use. While the specific behavior is not a direct result of using drugs, drug use may alter its frequency or seriousness. For example, some incarcerated alcoholics may need treatment when their drug use places other inmates or staff at risk. Even so, this treatment would be considered to be a "last resort," invoked only when other interventions, such as prohibiting alcohol use, have failed.

Regardless of the specific type of intervention, or the underlying circumstances necessitating it, privacy-intruding interventions are justifiable only when stringent conditions are met. These conditions require that an intervention be the least intrusive, least restrictive, and likely to be effective means reasonably available to avoid or minimize the harm that would result in the absence of the intervention. This approach is consonant with government responses to other risks inherent in daily life. Examples include requiring people to wear helmets while cycling to use seatbelts or babyseats when riding in automobiles, to obey speed limits and parking restrictions, to avoid littering, and to submit breathalyzer or other drug testing. In addition, individuals infected with certain communicable diseases must occasionally subject themselves to examination and treatment, or restrict their activity that places others at risk. Examples of government intervention in such situations include the treatment of syphillis or tuberculosis, the prohibition on obtaining employment as a food handler when carrying salmonella, and the exclusion of students from school when they are infectious with chickenpox or measles.

As in any situation that could give rise to state intervention, drug users need realistic opportunities to freely discuss their drug use and its attendant problems. Similarly, it is important that drug users have access to assistance without fear of self-incrimination, condemnation, or other harmful consequences from such disclosure. Thus, drug users must be able to openly seek advice, counsel, and care, especially when the drug user is prone to compulsive or harmful drug use. Unfortunately, the severe stigma associated with drug use, its widespread disapproval, and its illegality, can impede drug users from seeking this help. Too often, help is sought long after dependence has developed. Consequently, increasing the availability of such help and destigmatizing drug use are essential health interventions. This would include interventions aimed at stopping stereotypical responses against drug users, particularly those interventions that interfere with the access of drug users to these services, the protection of their privacy, and safeguarding the confidentiality of information about them.

3. DRUG TRAFFICKING

Trafficking in drugs presents a difficult dilemma regarding state intervention aimed at controlling drug use. Controlling drug use and suppressing drug trafficking can have devastating consequences for drug users when the supply of drugs is reduced without a corresponding reduction in demand. As long as the marketing and possession of drugs are prohibited, obtaining drugs will be a clandestine activity. This situation is problematic because it exposes a drug user, who might otherwise be considered innocent, to an illegal, profit-mad, crime-prone milieu. This scenario drives people seeking drugs underground to engage in illegal activity without any assurance of the purity of the black market commodity they buy. As a result, drug users purchase impure or adulterated drugs of unknown toxicity and potency, all the while facing arrest prosecution and imprisonment.

Additionally, suppressing the supply of drugs raises drug prices. This, in turn, favors trafficking in drugs by drug users to pay for their drug use. Substantial profits from the illegal sale of drugs, as well as "pyramiding,"[30] often entices (or drives) people, especially young people, to traffic in drugs. The profits favor market expansion, increasing the demand for drugs. The result is especially troubling when drug trafficking preys upon people, especially the young, prone to experiment with drugs though unaware of, unprepared for, or unable to prevent or minimize the risks associated with drug use. As a recent editorial in *The Economist* stated:

> The attitudes of most electorates and governments is to deplore the problems that the illegal drug trade brings, view the whole matter with distaste, and sit on the status quo – a policy of crime to which some addicts resort to finance their habits, and in which suppliers of illegal drugs habitually engage, exacts its price in victims' lives, not just money. The illegal trade in drugs supports organized crime the world over. It pulls drug-takers into a world of filthy needles, poisoned doses and pushers bent upon selling them more addictive and dangerous fixes.[31]

Efforts to prevent or stop trafficking are costly. Wider appreciation of the ineffectiveness and economic deficiencies of attempts to control drug use, primarily by suppressing the possession of and trafficking in drugs, has prompted some governments to reexamine or modify their control over the use of drugs, such as tobacco, alcohol, and cannabis. In some instances, governments have substituted regulatory controls, such as taxation and licensing approaches, for criminal justice measures. For instance:

> The most extreme example of alcohol control is total prohibition of alcoholic beverages, when the frequency of legal outlets is reduced to zero. There can be little doubt that during the first few

years of prohibition in Canada, Finland, and the United States, all indicators of alcohol consumption and alcohol problems reached their lowest level yet achieved in any period for which there are relevant data. It is also clear that in later years – say roughly 1923–1933 in the United States – as illegal trade became well established and the speakeasy and other clandestine outlets made their appearance, consumption increased substantially.

Between the world wars, total prohibition, however, turned out not to be viable in any of the western countries where it was tried. Deeply rooted traditional drinking patterns, sizeable economic interests in the production and trade of alcoholic beverages, and the governmental need for alcohol revenue, exacerbated by the Depression, led to the demise of prohibition and a general weakening of protemperance sentiments. Nevertheless, it was these historical processes which led to present-day governmental controls on alcohol, most pronounced in northern Europe, North America, and the Soviet Union.[32]

It is unlikely that either criminal suppression of drug possession or interventions aimed at reducing the demand for drugs, alone, could effectively control drug use and its harms. Accordingly, these two approaches must be balanced to eliminate or reduce both the highly profitable, crime-prone black market economy and the demand for drugs. Thus, there has been increased questioning and review of current legal and public policy responses to drug use to find a better balance among these alternatives. Suggestions as to the best balance among these alternatives is beyond the scope of this Article. However, in addressing this issue in the context of human rights, this Article points out the salience of human rights concepts and principles to help formulate and assess this balance.

4.REEVALUATION OF LEGAL AND POLICY RESPONSES TO DRUG USE

In many countries, there is a growing appreciation that legal and public policy responses to drug use may be made more effective, more productive, less costly, and less harmful. There is also an increasing momentum to reexamine the legal and public policy responses to drug use, particularly those aimed at preventing or reducing the harms brought about by drug trafficking and by the prohibition of the possession and use of many drugs. There is wide disagreement as to the proper approach to prevent and reduce these harms. This debate is highly polarized with proponents or increased efforts to suppress drug use on one side and proponents of removal or relaxation of drug controls on the other side. A recent statement by former U.S. Surgeon General Jocelyn Elders illustrates this controversy. The Surgeon General's remarks were reported in *The New York Times* as follows:

> I do feel that we would markedly reduce our crime rate if drugs were legalized. ... But I don't know all of the ramifications of this. I do feel that we need to do some studies. And in some of the countries that have legalized drugs and made it legal, they certainly have shown that there has been a reduction in their crime rate and there has been no increase in their drug use rate.[33]

Her statement was "met with a resounding chorus of dissociation and condemnation,"[34] including by White House officials. As a commentary, also published in *The New York Times*, noted:

> Dr. Elder's comments revived a perennial debate about the most effective way to handle the nation's drug problems. In the past few years a small but growing number of former and present government officials, commentators, and academics have argued that the present policy of aggressively prosecuting drug sellers and users should be reconsidered. They have compared the current state of drug policy to the prohibition of alcohol earlier this century and have said that the abolition of drug laws would eliminate the profit motive, the gangs, and the drug dealers.[35]

As the controversy regarding the Surgeon General's statements illustrate, opinions about what can and should be done to control drug use are not only polarized, but also entrenched. At one extreme are proponents of prohibition and drug interdiction who confront proponents of unfettered liberty and unrestricted access to drugs. In the middle ground are people working for incremental or gradual changes in drug control. These moderates are accelerating the momentum of harm reduction, prevention, and treatment approaches. Recently, an editorial in *The Lancet* described the debate:

> In a free society prohibition of intoxicants does not work. When such a policy was applied to alcohol in the USA it failed dismally; applied to heroin the outcome has been a disaster on a national and even international scale. Why should a counterproductive measure be pursued in the face of the evidence?
>
> Much has been invested in the war against drugs. Apart from the money, some reputations and many jobs depend on it; even if the chances of getting any of this investment back are remote, the war must go on. Also, it is felt that if it were not for the effort now being expended in this battle, the whole population might succumb to drug-taking and civilisation would crumble into anarchic groups of locust eaters.[36]

The editorial goes to point out that the middle ground often tends to be disregarded or overlooked in situations such as this, where opinions are so polarized, long-standing, and robust. In this setting, neither side can give up nor compromise their position or even acknowledge that there are alternatives which may resolve the dispute. To a great extent, this occurs when the stakes in the dispute are seen as too high or reputation may be lost in acknowledging alternative responses to drug use. Meanwhile, middle ground approaches, like those of harm reduction and public health, are impeded and cannot flourish. This is illustrated by a recent Australian government study which concluded that:

> The current debate over drug policy is largely over whether or not these costs are larger than those associated with heroin use itself and to what extent use would in fact increase in the absence of controls (and whether or not the *pattern* of use, even if more people used, would produce greater social costs in a less regulated

environment). For the most part the debate in the US has not addressed these issues in depth. Those who argue for changes to the status quo list the drawbacks of prohibitionism, but usually do not advance detailed or costed (in both financial and social senses) proposals for specific changes and only assert that the pattern of use would be less costly in the changed circumstances. The defenders of current policies, on the other hand, deliberately confuse drug use costs with drug control ones, use moralistic rhetoric to attack the critics, and merely assert that things would be worse under any more liberal drug control regime. The debate on both sides is long on invective, blurring of the issues and specious use of statistics, and short on reason, open-mindedness and facts.[37]

In this setting, public debate – free of rhetoric, ideology, and expediency – is needed. The first step in resolving this dispute is the recognition that controlling drug use and its harms can be improved. This requires examining opinions and options other than one's own. For example, this debate could begin with proposals, such as those of Nadelman and Wenner that are consonant with the promotion and protection of both respect for the human rights and the health of drug users and the public.

Any good nonprohibitionist policy has to contain three central ingredients. First, possession of small amounts of any drug for personal use has to be legal. Second, there have to be legal means by which adults can obtain drugs of certified quality, purity and quantity. These ways can vary from state to state and town to town, with the Federal Drug Administration playing a supervisory role in controlling quality, providing information and assuring truth in advertising. And third, citizens have to be empowered in their decisions about drugs. Doctors have a role in all this, but let's not give them all the power.

A drug policy with these ingredients would decimate the black market for drugs and take out of the hands of drug lords the 50 billion to 60 billion dollars in profits they earn each year. The nation would gain billions of dollars in law-enforcement savings and tax revenues, which could then be used to treat America's most serious problem: the miserable life prospects of millions of poor, undereducated Americans growing up in decaying, crime-ridden inner cities.[38]

Proposals such as this should not be viewed as a rejection of prohibition (which, undoubtedly, they are), but rather as an opening gambit with which to explore ways to more effectively control drug use and prevent or minimize its harms, while ensuring respect for the human rights of everyone.

5. HUMAN RIGHTS IMPLICATIONS OF A PRIVACY-BASED APPROACH TO DRUG USE

A privacy-based, autonomy emphasizing approach to drug use can have at least two important and potentially beneficial outcomes for drug users in relation to their opportunities to exercise their human rights. First, this approach would help to destigmatize drug use and drug users, thereby helping to decrease the exclusion of drug users and subsequent discrimination against them. Second, it would decrease human rights infringements resulting from some of the present efforts to interdict drugs by shifting emphasis from the control of drugs to the reduction of risks and the prevention of harms from drug use. There would also be additional benefits for drug users and for others. The criminal justice and prison systems would benefit by being able to focus their efforts at better controlling traffic in drugs. The health care system would benefit from the reduction in medical harms associated with drug use. Society would benefit by recovering otherwise lost opportunities to address the conditions underlying the vulnerability of some persons to use drugs and of drug users to be deprived of their human rights. Most importantly, drug users would benefit from the improved access to education, employment, housing counselling, support, and care. These changes would decrease the incidence of human rights infringements by reducing the number of drug users involved with the police, courts, prisons, and health care institutions. Lastly, increased respect for the human rights of drug users would extend to the communities to which drug users belong. This "vertical" effect of human rights would involve a spectrum of institutions and businesses, as well as individuals.[39]

NOTES

[1] Privacy may be viewed as "a right not to be interfered with." (Parent WA: III. Recent work on the concept of prvacy. *Am Phil Quart* 1983; 20:341-355; Richards DAJ: *Sex, Drugs, Death and the Law: An Essay on Human Rights and Overcriminalization*, Rowman & Littlefield, Totowa NJ, 1982, pp 34-35, with regard to drug use see Richards DAJ *ibid.* at pp 185-189. As the author has noted, privacy is a legal concept of recent origin. In medieval times, the individual was considered a member of a group, and the law was more concerned with defining status common to members of groups than with protection of individuality. Privacy as a legal concept could emerge only with legal recognition of the person as a democratically entitled, civilly responsible subject of rights, and this definition of the person is perhaps no more than two centuries old. Privacy remains imperfectly protected at law, however, because courts and legislators have been reluctant to accord privacy the protection accorded to other interests of the person. (Glen HP, Gilmore N, Somerville MA, Morissette Y-M: *HIV Infection, AIDS and Privacy. A Working Paper.* Montreal QC, McGill Centre for Medicine, Ethics and Law, March 1990, at pp 24-26). See also Mohr RD: Why sex is private: gays and police. *Public Affairs Q* 1987; 1:57-81, at p 57.

[2] This is illustrated by the deterrent to health care which can result when the transmission of a sexually transmitted disease is an express criminal offence: With respect to destigmatization in the context of STDs, in particular AIDS, it is interesting to note that in 1985 the Canadian Parliament revoked the section in the *Criminal Code* of Canada that expressly made it an offence to transmit an STD. One aim in doing this could have been to ensure that fear of criminal liability would not deter persons from seeking counsel or treatment in relation to AIDS. This section of the *Criminal Code* had been enacted in 1919, "as part of used in only one prosecution, in 1926. This repeal does not mean that persons cannot be held criminally liable in Canada for transmission of HIV – they can and have been, in particular, under general criminal law provisions that include aggravated assault, attempting to cause bodily harm, criminal negligence (showing wanton or reckless indifference to human life or safety), and common nuisance. [references omitted] (Gilmore N, Somerville MA: Stimatization, scapegoating, and discrimination in sexually transmitted diseases: overcoming "them" and "us". *Soc Science Med* 1994, p 1343.

[3] Some of the impairments directly attributable to drug use include: demotivation and disregard for the user's own health (especially when there is intense compulsive drug use); prolonged craving and withdrawl disorders; impaired memory function from chronic LSD use; vasculitis and ischemic disorders (such as myocardial infarction from cocaine use and severe depression following its use); neurological disorders associated with alcohol use (such as neuropathy, cerebellar degeneration, and Korsakoff's syndrome); and lung cancer and chronic obstructive pulmonary disease from tobacco smoking. See Schuckit MA: Alcohol and alcoholism. In (Wilson JD, Braunwald E, Isselfbacher KJ, Petersdorf RG, Martin JB, Fauci AS Root RK (eds): *Harrison's*

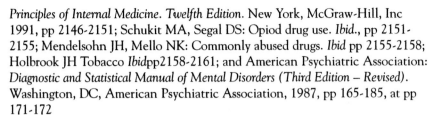

Principles of Internal Medicine. Twelfth Edition. New York, McGraw-Hill, Inc 1991, pp 2146-2151; Schukit MA, Segal DS: Opiod drug use. *Ibid.*, pp 2151-2155; Mendelsohn JH, Mello NK: Commonly abused drugs. *Ibid* pp 2155-2158; Holbrook JH Tobacco *Ibid* pp2158-2161; and American Psychiatric Association: *Diagnostic and Statistical Manual of Mental Disorders (Third Edition – Revised).* Washington, DC, American Psychiatric Association, 1987, pp 165-185, at pp 171-172

[4] For a discussion of disability in international law, see Despouy L: *Human Rights and Disabled Persons.* (Study Series 6). Geneva, U.N. Centre for Human Rights, 1993 [UN Publication Sale No E 92.XIV.4], and in the law of the United States, see Parmet WE: Discrimination and disability: the challenges of the ADA. *Law Med Health Care;* 18: 331-344

[5] In the context of American disability law, see Henderson Jr RP: Addiction as disability: the protection of alcoholics and drug addicts under the Americans with Disabilities Act of 1990. *Vanderbilt LJ* 1991; 44:713-744

[6] Slivis J, Hendriks A, Gilmore N (eds): *Drug Use and Human Rights In Europe. Report from the European Commission.* Utrecht, NL. Willem Pompe Institute for Criminal Law & Criminology, Faculty of Law, Utrecht University, 1992

[7] Schoman F: AIDS and privacy. In (Reamer FG, ed) *AIDS and Ethics.* New York NY, Columbia University Press, 1991, pp 240-276, at pp 242-243.

[8] Art. 17.1 of the *International Covenant on Civil and Political Rights* states that, "No one shall be subjected to arbitrary or unlawful Interference with his privacy, family, home or correspondence, not to unlawful acts on his honour or reputation."

[9] For a discussion of autonomy with regard to human rights, see Richards DAJ: *Sex, Drugs, Death and the Law: An Essay on Human Rights and Overcriminalization.* Rowman & Littlefield, Totowa, NJ 1982, at pp 8-9 and Husak DN: *Drugs and Rights.* Cambridge University Press, NY 1992m at pp 100-117

[10] The term "excessive" has been chosen to recognize that there is probably no human decision or activity which does not have consequences on others, including society in general. These consequences may be beneficial or harmful or both, and direct or indirect or both. Drug use is *not* considered to be excessive when its benefits for the user and others outweigh its harms, and when its harms do not exceed those which can result from other private and voluntary activities, such as playing sports, leisure activities, reading, having an occasional drink, etc. When the harms from drug use are not judged to be "excessive" by both of these criteria, then it can be considered to be an "innocuous" activity. Before there is a continuum of drug use, ranging from occasional or experimental drug use to life-imperiling compulsive use, and because benefits and harms can vary depending on the drug used, the user, and the setting in which it is used, it is not possible to demarcate precisely when drug use may or may not become innocuous. Generally, however, drug use is likely to be innocuous by these criteria when it is not persistent and especially when it is not compulsive. This is reflected in the distinction that is often made between drug use and drug abuse.

[11] BMA Professional and Scientific Division : *Living with Risk. The British*

Medical Association Guide. Chichester UK, J Wiley and Sons, 1987, in particular pp 95-105

[12] Public morality, reflecting a moral inadequacy model of drug use, is often claimed as a basis to condemn and drug use.

[13] Winick C: Social behavior, public policy, and nonharmful drug use. *Millband Q* 1991; 69 (3): 437-459

[14] Eisenhandler J, Drucker E: Opiate dependency among the subscribers of a New York area private insurance plan. *J Am Med Assoc* 1993; 269: 2890-2891.

[15] Gold MS, Schuchard K, Gleaton T: Correspondence: LSD use among US high school students. *J Am Med Assoc* 1994; 271: 426-427

[16] Shah CP: *Public Health and Preventative Medicine in Canada*. Toronto, Univ of Toronto Press, 1994, at p 90

[17] *Ibid.*

[18] For a discussion of privacy see Meyers DT: *Self, Society, and Personal Choice*. New York, NY Columbia University Press, 1989

[19] See the discussion on privacy *supra* note 1 and Mitchell CN: A justice based argument for the uniform regulation of psychoactive drugs. *McGill L J* 1986: 31: 213-263. See also Bakalar JB, Ginspoon L: *Drug Control in a Free Society*. New York, Cambridge University Press 1984, at pp 118-119

[20] Solomon RM: Canada's federal drug legislation. In Blackwell JC, Erickson PG (eds) *Illicit Drugs in Canada*. Nelson Canada, Scarborough ON, 1988, at p 216

[21] *Ib id*, at p 216

[22] Husak DN: *Drugs and Rights*. Cambridge University Press, New York, 1992.

[23] Friedelbaum SH: *Human Rights in the States. New Directions in Constitutional Policy Making*. New York NY, Greenwood Press, 1988, at p 77, citing Ravin v. State, 537 P.2d 494, 509 (Alas. 1975)

[24] Ten Have HAMJ: Drug addiction, society and health care ethics. In (Gillon R, ed) *Principles of Health Care Ethics*. London, John Wiley & Sons, 1994, pp 895-902, at 900-902

[25] See eg Caudill BD, Hoffman JA, Hubbard RL: Parental history of substance abuse as a risk factor in predicting crack smokers' substance use, illegal activities, and psychiatric status. *Am J Drug Alcohol Abuse* 1994; 20: 341-354. Hawk M, Norton A: How social policies make matters worse: the case of maternal substance abuse. *J Drug Issues* 1994; 24: 517-526.

[26] Denison J: The efficacy and constitutionality of criminal punishment for maternal substance abuse. *S Calif L Rev* 1991; 64; 1104-41

[27] Nurco DN, Balter MB, Kinlock T: Vulnerability to narcotic addiction: preliminary findings. *J Drug Issues* 1994; 24: 293-314

[28] For an example of this approach, see Garrett L: *The Coming Plague. Newly Emerging Diseases in a World Out of Balance*. New York NY, Farrar, Strauss and Giroux, 1994, at p 280

[29] Bayer R: *Private Acts, Social Consequences. AIDS and the Politics of Public Health*. New Brunswick, NJ, Rutgers University Press, 1989.

[30] Smart RG, Adalf EM, Walsh GM: Adolescent drug sellers: trends, characteristics and profiles. *Br J Addict* 1992; 82: 1561-1570; Fields AB: Weedslingers: young black marijuana dealers. In Beschner G, Friedman AS

(eds) *Teen Drug Use*. Toronto ON, Lexington Books, 1986, pp 85-104.

[31] *The Economist* 15 May 1993, at p 13

[32] Osterberg E: Current approaches to limit alcohol abuse and the negative consequences of use: A comparative overview of available options and an assessment of proven effectiveness. In Aasland OG: *Expert Meeting on The Negative Social Consequences of Alcohol Use, Oslo, 27-31 August 1990*. Oslo, Norwegian Ministry of Health and Social Affairs, 1991, pp 266-199, at p 278

[33] Kaplan HI, Saddock BJ, Grebb JA : *Kaplan and Saddock's Synopsis of Psychiatry, Behavioral Sciences, Clinical Psychiatry*. Baltimore, MD, Williams & Wilkins, 1994, at p 383.

[34] Jonas S: Dealing with the drug problem. *Preventive Med* 1994; 23: 539-544, at 539

[35] Kaplan HI, Saddock BJ, Grebb JA *supra* note 33, at p 383

[36] Anonymous: Editorial. Of auctions, dilemmas, and models of escalation behaviour. *Lancet* 1989; ii, 1487-1488.

[37] Wardlaw G: Overview of national drug control strategies. In National Campaign Against Drug Abuse: *Comparative Analysis of Illicit Drug Strategy*. Canberra, Australian Government Publishing Service, 1992, at p 13 [emphasis in the original]

[38] Nadelman E, Wenner JS: Toward a sane national drug policy. *Rolling Stone 5* May 1994, pp 26-28, at pp 27-28

[39] van Banning TRG: *Human Rights reference Handbook*. Den Haag NL, Netherlands Ministry of Foreign Affairs, 1992, p 3.

DEBATE QUESTIONS

1.The author divides this selection into four main sections: privacy; human rights; impairment of health and autonomy of drug users; and discrimination. Oftentimes in debate you might choose to follow all of the arguments presented and respond to each in turn or you might address the issues you find most relevant. If you were to choose one or two of these issues, which would they be? Which arguments do you find the most persuasive and why?

2. In the section of this book that addressed human rights, personal liberty was an important consideration. In this article personal liberty, or autonomy, plays a big role. The following sentence helps focus the issue: 'This leads to the questions of whether or not voluntary innocuous drug use can be distinct from such activities with regard to their benefits, risks and harms.' How would you answer this question?

3.Personal privacy goes hand-in-hand with personal liberty. And the issue of drug use can be portrayed – as it is in this article – as an issue of personal privacy. Few would claim, though, that personal privacy is absolute. Where does the author weigh in on the issue of privacy? Do you find his arguments persuasive?

Clinical progress and the future of HIV exceptionalism[1]

by Ronald Bayer, PhD,
Division of Sociomedical Sciences, Columbia University

Since HIV was first discovered twenty years ago, there is now more knowledge available about the infection and its modes of transmission, and the panic and fear that were associated with the early years of the epidemic have passed. In some countries there is treatment available to effectively stop the progression of the disease and allow people infected with the virus to live a life of anyone with any other chronic illness. These achievements would have been impossible without scientific progress and the exceptional attitude towards HIV/AIDS. The crucial therapeutic changes may entail an inevitable change in policy. Why should HIV/AIDS be treated exceptionally now, when there are obvious benefits to the early detection of the infection? Has the time come to reassess HIV's exceptional status and treat it like any other disease? If so, should "HIV exceptionalism" be fully discarded, or would it be better to just limit it? Possible scenarios and consequences of treating HIV/AIDS like any other disease are demonstrated with regards to screening of pregnant women and newborns, name reporting and access to health care.

I t is a remarkable feature of the epidemic's first years that in virtually every economically advanced democratic nation, a determination was made to approach AIDS differently from other
major infectious threats and sexually transmitted diseases.

The decision entailed a commitment to rely on prevention measures that were noncoercive – that respected the privacy and social
rights of those who were at risk. Mass education, voluntary testing,
and counseling were at the center of a public health strategy that
sought to avoid interventions that might "drive the epidemic
underground." Gay leaders and AIDS activists played a crucial role
in shaping these policies, which were endorsed by public health
officials, medical professionals, and a broad array of political actors,
all the more remarkable because the epidemic's early years coincid-
ed with the commencement of the conservative politics of the
Reagan era.[2]

In 1991, the term "HIV exceptionalism" was proposed to distinguish the policies that had emerged in the face of the AIDS epidemic from more conventional approaches to public health threats.
The notion of exceptionalism was put forward at a time when epidemiological and clinical changes were already undermining the
alliance of forces that had fostered its emergence, when a process of
normalization had begun:

> "As AIDS becomes less threatening, the claims of those who
> argued that the exceptional threat would require exceptional
> policies have begun to lose their force. The most important factor
> in accounting for the changing contours of public health policy,
> however, has been the notable advances in therapeutic prospects.
> The possibility of managing HIV-related opportunistic infections
> and the hopes of slowing the course of HIV progression itself
> have increased the importance of early identification of those

with HIV infection. That, in turn, has produced a willingness to consider traditional public health approaches to screening, reporting, and partner notification."[3]

It is now 8 years since those words were written, and the time is ripe to examine the fate of exceptionalism in America with a discussion of 3 issues: HIV testing of newborns and pregnant women, the reporting by name of those with HIV to public health registries, and access to care on the part of those infected with HIV. In so doing, it will be possible to demonstrate how the exceptionalist perspective, which emerged at a time of therapeutic impotence, has been subject to increasingly aggressive challenges as therapeutic prospects have improved. Such an analysis represents a contribution to the understanding of the ways in which medicine, science, and politics interact in the framing of public health policy more generally.

Debates about testing are not new, as anyone familiar with the confrontations over sickle cell[4] and neonatal[5] screening will readily appreciate. Conflicts over reporting to public health registries are as old as the practice itself, as the reporting of cases of tuberculosis[6] and of syphilis[7] makes clear. Unique medical entitlements play a special safety-valve role in a health care system that fails to provide universal protection against the cost of illness, as the history of the end-stage renal disease[8] and black lung programs attests.[9]

SCREENING NEWBORNS AND PREGNANT WOMEN

Since the HIV-antibody test was introduced in 1985, it has been the subject of intense debate. Fear about how those identified as having HIV might be subject to discrimination and stigma; concern about how the diagnosis of HIV infection, in the absence of effective therapy, could produce unbearable psychological burdens; and a belief that testing had little to do with behavioral change led AIDS activists generally, and gay leaders specifically, to adopt a posture of hostility and/or skepticism regarding the test.[10] On the other hand, many public health officials believed that the identification of infected persons could play a crucial role in fostering mass behavioral change. Out of their confrontations emerged a broad consensus that, except in a few well-defined circumstances, people should be tested only with their informed, voluntary, and specific consent.

As a result of clinical developments – the belief that treatment with zidovudine for those with CD4+ cell counts of less than 500x106 /L could delay the onset of symptomatic AIDS and the recognition of the importance of primary prophylaxis against Pneumocystis carinii pneumonia-by 1990, the medical significance of identifying those with early HIV disease had become clear. Consequently, the clinical and political context of the debate about testing underwent a fundamental change. Gay organizations began to urge homosexual and bisexual men to have their antibody status determined under confidential or anonymous conditions.[11] Physicians pressed for AIDS to be incorporated into the medical mainstream and for the HIV-antibody test to be treated like other blood tests – ie, given with the presumed consent of the patient.[12]

The movement toward routine or mandatory testing has been especially pronounced in the case of pregnant women and newborns. Despite that the actual infection status of antibody-positive newborns could not be determined because all infants born to infected mothers carry maternal antibodies, and despite the absence in the late 1980s of a specific therapeutic intervention for such asymptomatic infants, several pediatricians – notably those who were responsible for the care of newborns with AIDS-became strong advocates for the early identification of newborns who might carry HIV. Thus, with a sense of urgency, Scott et al wrote in 1989,

"There is only a short period during which antiviral treatment or other effective prophylactic measures can be initiated before the onset of clinical disease. This emphasizes the importance of early recognition of HIV-1 infection in children to permit early and effective treatment."[13]

To the extent that this perspective was linked to calls for mandatory screening, it was met with profound resistance. Opponents of mandatory testing of newborns asserted that coercive strategies not only would provide little benefit to possibly infected children but also would entail compulsory identification of infection in the (typically minority) mothers – a violation of their privacy rights.[14] Progress in the next years was to make it possible to determine whether HIV-positive newborns were truly infected soon after birth,[15] and the improved prospects of clinical management were to make such determinations appear all the more critical.[16] So it is not surprising that pediatricians were to become increasingly impatient with the strict regimen of explicit and specific consent that surrounded the testing of newborns for HIV[17] all the more striking because routine and unconsented testing of newborns for inborn errors of metabolism such as phenylketonuria was mandated in virtually every state.

Ultimately, in late spring 1993, New York State, which together with California had pioneered the enactment of stringent informed consent requirements for HIV testing, seriously considered legislation that would have mandated the screening of newborns for HIV infection.[18,19] It was to provoke a cry of outrage from the advocates of women's rights and other defenders of exceptionalism. The proposed amendment to the state's testing policy was introduced into the New York State Assembly by Nettie Myersohn, a liberal Democrat with a history of support for reproductive rights. Focusing on the risk that infected women could transmit HIV to their uninfected infants through breast-feeding and the prospect that initiating early therapeutic intervention could enhance the life prospects of already-infected newborns, she challenged the morality of the state's ongoing blinded seroprevalence study of newborns that could identify the number of newborns who carried maternal antibody but could not, by definition, identify which newborns were potentially infected. In a press release, she declared, "It's a Baby, Not a Statistic, Stupid."

Stunningly, the proposed legislation won the support not only of the local newspaper, New York Newsday[20] but also 2 of the 3 New York branches of the American Academy of Pediatrics.[21] When, at last, The New York Times spoke out on the issue, it made clear how it believed the legislature should decide the issue:

> "No doubt privacy is vital for many AIDS campaigns. But in applying it to newborns, the experts are following their theology over a cliff.... From the evidence at hand, a strong case can be made for exempting newborns from the general policy of voluntary testing after informed consent. It seems cruel and is guided to protect parental privacy when the welfare of tiny babies is at stake."[22]

For those locked in conflict, the 1993 controversy in New York, with more HIV-infected newborns than any other state, represented a critical moment in the conflict over newborn testing. Were politically liberal New York to abandon its commitment to voluntarism, it might well set the stage for similar action in other jurisdictions. It was in large measure the extraordinary mobilization of women AIDS activists, who argued passionately that the pending legislation would represent an affront to the dignity and rights of black and Hispanic women and an unwarranted politicization of the practice of pediatrics that would threaten the well-being of women and children as well, that forestalled legislative approval.

Although this initial effort to mandate newborn testing was thwarted, in part because New York State's Commissioner of Health opposed the move as involving an unnecessary intrusion on maternal rights, the picture changed radically 3 years later. In 1996, with a new political administration in the state and a rapidly evolving clinical picture suggesting that early intervention was, indeed, crucial for infected newborns, the governor of New York, George Pataki, introduced legislation that would mandate newborn screening "to ensure that those who are born exposed to HIV receive prompt and immediate care and treatment that can enhance, prolong, and possibly save their lives."[23] With the support of his chief health official, Barbara De Buono, MD, and the organization representing New York's county health officials (New York State Association of County Health Officials, memorandum, March 15, 1995), the opposition to the proposed bill crumbled, and an overwhelming majority in both houses of the legislature voted for a measure that a few years earlier could not muster anything approaching the requisite support (1996 NY Laws, Chapter 220).

Ironically, the passage of the newborn testing legislation occurred at a time when interest had begun to shift to the question of screening pregnant women. Three pediatricians long associated with the care of newborns infected with HIV noted:

> "This is another example of scientific progress leaping over the stalled engines of public policy. The inescapable issue is that mothers should undergo testing for HIV infection during pregnancy, not that newborns should undergo testing after delivery [when it may already be too late to make the most significant difference]."[24]

The shift toward the question of maternal screening had begun in early 1994 as the result of the remarkable finding of clinical trial 076[25] that the administration of zidovudine during pregnancy could reduce the rate of vertical transmission by two thirds. Coming at a time when the general clinical picture surrounding antiretroviral therapy appeared gloomy and when prospects for a preventive vaccine seemed to be less than hopeful, these were striking findings. In the aftermath of the trial, pressure has mounted to ensure that infected women are identified early in pregnancy.

Although advocates on behalf of women's interests, including the American College of Obstetrics and Gynecology,[26] have fought hard to preserve the right of pregnant women to undergo HIV testing only after specific informed consent, the prospect of saving newborns from HIV infection provided the foundation for an assault on that posture. That routine or mandatory testing for hepatitis B and syphilis was a matter of policy and/or practice in many states made the exceptionalist demand for specific informed consent in the case of HIV seem increasingly anomalous. A survey[27] of California obstetricians done in the aftermath of clinical trial 076 found that 64% supported mandatory testing of pregnant women. Even some of those who had been long associated with the defense of the rights of pregnant women began to modify their position. Howard Minkoff, MD, an obstetrician in Brooklyn, NY, and Anne Willoughby, MD, of the National Institute of Child Health and Human Development suggested that the principle of informed consent should be supplanted with an "informed right of refusal." The purpose was clear. "When an informed right of refusal... is used... a psychological burden is shifted from those who would choose the test to those who would refuse."[28] Requiring a special effort to say no would dramatically increase the percentage of persons testing, they believed. Others[29] have called for the routinization of HIV testing during pregnancy, citing data that suggested that pregnant women themselves supported such a move. In 1998, the Institute of Medicine, in its report Reducing the Odds: Preventing Perinatal Transmission of HIV in the United States,[30] recommended the routine testing of all pregnant women in the United States, with an informed right of refusal. Reflective of the changes that have occurred, 2 members of the panel that made the recommendation had long opposed any deviation from the requirement of specific informed consent before testing for HIV.

More striking was the decision of the House of Delegates of the American Medical Association, which in June 1996 passed a resolution calling for mandatory testing of pregnant women. Commenting on that decision, a past president of the association said,

> "The Association opposed testing early on because society had little to offer victims of HIV other than discrimination. But now that we can offer treatment and alter the course of the disease, and hopefully prevent it in the unborn child, we can embrace a more scientifically oriented position that might benefit all."[31]

Finally, in that same year, the US Congress expressed its discontent with the requirement that the testing of pregnant women and newborns be based on specific informed consent. After a protracted battle over the reauthorization of the Ryan White Care Act (Public Law 104-147) – which supports local AIDS treatment efforts – the House and Senate endorsed an amendment that would require each state that received federal funds under the act to demonstrate that it had, by the year 2000, either achieved a 50% reduction in new pediatric AIDS cases, initiated a program of mandatory newborn screening, or attained a 95% testing rate of pregnant women (AIDS Policy Center Brief, May 22, 1996). Failure to reach those stringent goals would result in a loss of critically important federal funds. By establishing those targets, the federal government had all but dictated that the states impose mandatory screening either during pregnancy or for newborns.

The move toward mandatory screening represents a significant departure from the strictures of exceptionalism made possible in the cases of pregnant women and newborns by existing conventions that provided a warrant for prenatal and postnatal screening dictated by the interest of the children. Explicitly mandatory testing measures are less likely to be adopted for other clinical populations. Rather, the departure from exceptionalism will, in all likelihood, take the form of integrating HIV testing into clinical practice where the standards of consent for blood testing are less demanding than those informed by the exceptionalist perspective that emerged in the formative years of the AIDS epidemic.

REPORTING BY NAME

The early years of the epidemic were characterized by great fears about how the public's reaction to a new, lethal, and infectious disease would amplify existing antagonisms toward those who were thought to be at greatest risk – gay men, drug users, and their sexual partners. It is no surprise, therefore, that the need for confidentiality of the clinical records of those diagnosed as having AIDS took on such importance. It was required to protect vulnerable persons and was embraced by public health officials who understood that in the absence of stringent privacy protections, people might be reluctant to seek clinical care and counseling. (Exacting confidentiality requirements for vulnerable, even unpopular, populations is hardly new. Federal standards governing drug abuse-treatment centers were promulgated to foster the entry into treatment.)

Given those concerns, it is remarkable that little opposition existed in the epidemic's first years to making AIDS cases reportable by name to confidential state public health registries. AIDS activists appreciated that such reporting was crucial to the understanding of the epidemiology of the new disease.[2] The acceptance of AIDS-case reporting requirements was facilitated by the well-established record of state health departments in protecting such records from unwarranted disclosure. Since the inception of HIV testing, however, there has been sharp debate about whether the names of all infected persons, regardless of whether they had received an AIDS diagnosis, should be reported to state registries. Activists who accepted AIDS-case reporting opposed HIV reporting because of concerns about privacy, confidentiality, and discrimination.[2] Many public health officials opposed such a move because of the potential effect on the willingness of people to seek HIV testing and counseling.

On the other hand, early on, many public health officials did become strong advocates of HIV reporting. Their claims sought to underscore the extent to which the public health benefits of HIV reporting would be like those that followed from more broadly conceived reporting requirements – those that applied to syphilis, tuberculosis, and AIDS itself. Thus, in the mid-1980s, the director of the health department in Colorado, a low-prevalence state, declared that name reporting of HIV cases could ensure that people with HIV were properly counseled about preventing transmission of the virus, permit those charged with surveillance to better accomplish their tasks, and create the possibility of expeditiously notifying infected persons when effective treatments became available (Thomas Vernon, oral communication, November 14, 1986). Finally, name reporting for HIV cases was viewed as essential to an effective program of partner notification.

Such views had relatively little influence in high-prevalence states, although they provoked a sense of alarm among AIDS activists and their political allies, steeling them against any indication that states within which they were influential might follow suit.

As therapeutic advances began to emerge in the late 1980s, fissures began to appear in the relatively broad and solid alliance against named reporting. Thus, in 1989, Stephen Joseph, MD, New York City's Health Commissioner, stated[32] that the prospects of early clinical intervention warranted "a shift toward a disease-control approach to HIV infection along the lines of classic tuberculosis practices," including the "reporting of seropositives." Although his proposal met with fierce and effective resistance, it is clear that his call represented part of a national trend.

At the end of November 1990, the CDC declared its support for HIV reporting, which it asserted could "enhance the ability of local, state and national agencies to project the level of required resources" for care and prevention services.[33] Within a week, the House of Delegates of the American Medical Association endorsed the reporting of names as well, thus breaking with the traditional resistance of medical practitioners to such intrusions on the physician-patient relationship. In 1991, New Jersey became the first high-prevalence state to require HIV-case reporting by name.

In the following years, the CDC continued to press for named reporting of HIV cases, an effort that has now assumed the dimensions of a campaign. During the years, it was supported by a growing number of public health officials. Indeed, the Council of State and Territorial Epidemiologists adopted resolutions in 1989, 1991, 1993, and 1995 encouraging states to consider the implementation of HIV case surveillance (Council of State and Territorial Epidemiologists, unpublished data, 1997). Central to their argument was the assertion that AIDS-case reporting captured an epidemic that was as much as a decade old and that an accurate picture of the incidence and prevalence of HIV infection required a surveillance system based on HIV-case reporting.

Nevertheless, resistance on the part of AIDS activist organizations and their political allies persisted, and as a consequence, HIV cases typically became reportable by name only in states with relatively few cases of AIDS, which were typically states that did not have large cosmopolitan communities with effectively organized gay constituencies. By 1996, although 26 states had adopted HIV-case reporting, they represented jurisdictions with only 24% of reported AIDS cases.[34] By October 1998, the Figure hadrisen to 32 states (3 states reported only pediatric cases), involving about 33% of AIDS cases (CDC, unpublished data). Furthermore, it was clear that the hold of the exceptionalist perspective on reporting was weakening. Florida, with its large case load, had become a reporting state, and Texas, which together with Maryland, had experimented with a unique identifier system of HIV-case reporting as an alternative to the use of names, had come to the conclusion that such an approach was unworkable.[35]

Nothing more forcefully underscores the changes now occurring than the events that have transpired in New York. In 1997, the state with the largest concentration of AIDS cases began, for the first time, to consider name reporting. Although the state health department task force charged with the responsibility of advising the commissioner of health on the matter remained bitterly divided, the lines of cleavage were clear. It was only the representatives of community-based organizations who opposed name reporting.

Public health officials on the committee and throughout the state supported HIV-case reporting by name (Mark Rapoport, MD, oral communication, May 15, 1998). That deadlock only paved the way for final action in the legislative arena. On June 19, 1998, in the waning hours of the legislative session, the Democrat-controlled assembly voted 112 to 34 for a bill that would mandate case reporting by name and a more aggressive approach to partner notification. In so doing, it joined the Republican-dominated state senate, which had already passed the bill (1998 NY Laws, Chapter 163). For advocates of name reporting, the significance of the New York decision could not be overstated.

The New York decision is best understood in the effects of therapeutic advances on the national policy debate on name reporting. That effect is made clear in an editorial[36] published in late 1977. Jointly authored by Larry Gostin, a well-known proponent of civil liberties, John Ward, MD, of the CDC, and Cornelius Baker, the African American President of the National Association of People With AIDS, the editorial represented a new alliance. Locating the argument for named reporting in the context of the remarkable therapeutic achievements represented by the protease inhibitors and the advent of triple-combination antiretroviral therapy, the authors declared:

> "We are at a defining moment of the epidemic of HIV infection and AIDS. With therapy that delays the progression to AIDS, mental illnesses, and death, HIV infection or AIDS is becoming a complex clinical disease that does not lend itself to monitoring based on end stage illness. Unless we revise our surveillance system, health authorities will not have reliable information about the prevalence of HIV infection.... To correct these deficiencies, we propose that all states require HIV case reporting."[36]

Among the additional advantages of HIV-case reporting, it was asserted that it would give public health authorities a greater ability to "ensure timely referrals for health and social services."

Although many, if not most, AIDS-service organizations remain adamantly opposed to name reporting, arguing instead for the use of unique identifiers, the public health community, with the CDC in the lead, concluded that such an approach would simply impede the adoption of an effective system of surveillance. Strikingly, the proponents of name reporting for HIV cases now include the former executive director of the National Lesbian and Gay Task Force, Jeff Levi, and Michael Isbell, former policy director of the Gay Men's Health Crisis, the nation's largest AIDS-service organization. Both had played a central role in shaping the exceptionalist perspective within which name reporting of HIV cases had been anathema.

ACCESS TO CARE AND AMERICAN EXCEPTIONALISM

Although the unraveling of HIV exceptionalism has been largely driven by important clinical developments, the extent to which persons with HIV have been able to gain access to the new clinical achievements has been profoundly affected by a different kind of exceptionalism. America stands alone among advanced industrial democracies in failing to guarantee access to medical care regardless of ability to pay. More than 40 million Americans have no health insurance. Millions more are inadequately insured. The picture has deteriorated since the collapse of President Clinton's health reform initiative.

This, then, was the context in which the medical needs of people with HIV disease had to be met. Some had private insurance, those who became impoverished because of their disease often qualified for Medicaid,[37] but many remained unprotected. To meet their needs, special programs were developed. The federal government, through the Ryan White Care Act, directed hundreds of millions of dollars to localities to provide medical services. Among the initiatives under the act was the AIDS Drug Assistance Program (ADAP), designed to pay for AIDS-related medicines. But the patchwork effort was never adequate and left many without needed protection. When the protease inhibitors emerged and combination antiretroviral therapy became the standard of care, the system was strained to the limits. Medication costs alone for those receiving care could range from $10,000 to $15,000 a year.[38] One early review of dramatically improved therapeutic prospects added the disheartening caveat that the new achievements were important "at least for those socioeconomically privileged."[39]

In the period since the protease inhibitors became available, ADAP has experienced persistent shortfalls in funding. As a result, various rationing strategies have been used. At one point, nearly half of the ADAP programs limited access to protease inhibitors.[40] In 1996, the coordinator of Oregon's program explained that such coverage "would blow our budget out of the water."[41] A 1998 report[42] by the National ADAP Monitoring Project found that 15 states maintained waiting lists for entry to ADAP or for access to protease inhibitors. North Carolina, which had no formal waiting list, had simply stopped authorizing new clients for its ADAP. Only 2 state programs covered the 14 drugs strongly recommended by the Public Health Service for the prevention of opportunistic infections.

It is a remarkable paradox that the (costly) therapeutic achievements that have rendered the exceptionalist perspective so vulnerable have set the stage for challenging the programs that seek to ensure – however inadequately – access to those same treatments. Casarett and Lantos[43] assert:

"The absence of [benefits like those in the Ryan White Act] for persons with other stigmatizing diseases is troubling. We believe that this discrepancy leaves AIDS exceptionalism vulnerable to the accusation of injustice."[43]

Within this context, a surprising challenge to exceptionalism emerged from within the AIDS activist community. Martin Delaney, the founder of Project Inform, a community-based organization in San Francisco, Calif, thus stated: "There are certainly other life-threatening diseases out there. Some of them kill a lot more people than AIDS does. So in one sense, it is almost an advantage to be HIV positive. It makes no sense."[44]

This challenge to exceptionalism does not represent a mainstream position within the AIDS activist community. Nevertheless, it reflects a sense of disquiet. What can explain this willingness to argue against the advantages of exceptionalism? The answer can perhaps be found in the decision of the Clinton Administration not to ensure universal protection for all poor persons with HIV disease.[45] After a long period of deliberation, the administration declared that such an effort would not be "budget-neutral." Given the requirements of deficit reduction – the central goal of the American political system at this juncture – that was no longer acceptable. In addition, it was argued that to provide people with HIV infection guaranteed health insurance protection while others did not have it would raise "ethical concerns."

Thus, Delaney's challenge may reflect a sense that the pressing medical needs of people infected with HIV were no longer adequate for asserting a unique right to costly medical services. Only by broadening the political constituency for ensuring access to medical care could the needs of people infected with HIV be secured.

CONCLUSIONS

The advances of medicine have served to undermine the exceptionalism of the HIV epidemic's first years in America. Practices uniquely informed by a commitment to privacy rights are increasingly vulnerable to challenge as despair and therapeutic impotence give way to a (perhaps premature) therapeutic triumphalism. Restrictions on access to costly therapeutic advances have underscored the limits of exceptionalism as a way of meeting the medical needs of those with HIV disease in a health care system characterized by profound inequities. It is not the provision of special medical entitlement to those with a fatal viral infection that renders them ethically problematical. Rather, it is the failure to extend medical protection to all in need that represents the ethical affront. The provision of even expensive medical care to 1 group in America should not affect the claims of others in need. Under prevailing economic conditions, the allocation of health care need not be a zero-sum game. Nevertheless, the uniqueness of AIDS benefits renders them politically vulnerable. The interests of those with HIV infection are thus bound to those with other diseases. Only a system that guarantees access to care to all in medical need, regardless of their ability to pay, will in the long run protect the needs of those infected with HIV.

That the era of exceptionalism may be coming to a close is, thus, not the end of the story. The privacy interests of persons infected with HIV requires a basic encounter with the role and limits of medical privacy, more generally, just as the need for HIV care requires a confrontation with the broader question of justice in the American health care system.

NOTES

1. Rosenberg PS, Biggar RJ. Trends in HIV incidence among young adults in the United States. JAMA. 1998;279:1894-1899.
2. Bayer R. Private Acts Social Consequences: AIDS and the Politics of Public Health. New York, NY: Free Press; 1989.
3. Bayer R. Public health policy and the AIDS epidemic: an end to HIV exceptionalism? N Engl J Med. 1991;324:1500-1504.
4. Bergsma D. Ethical, Social and Legal Dimensions of Screening for Human Genetic Disease. Miami, Fla: Symposia Specialists; 1974.
5. Faden RR, Holtzman NA, Chwalow AJ. Parental rights, child welfare, and public health: the case of PKU screening. Am J Public Health. 1982;72:1396-1400.
6. Fox D. From TB to AIDS: value conflicts in reporting. Hastings Cent Rep. 1986;16(suppl):11-16.
7. Brandt A. No Magic Bullet. New York, NY: Oxford University Press; 1987.
8. Rettig RA. Health Care Technology: Lessons Learned From the End-Stage Renal Disease Experience. Santa Monica, Calif: RAND; November 1976:1-36. The RAND Paper Series, Publication P-5820.
9. Seltzer C. Moral dimensions of occupational health: the case of the 1969 Coal Mine Health and Safety Act. In: Bayer R. The Health and Safety of Workers. New York, NY: Oxford University Press; 1988:242-270.
10. Don't take the test. New York Native. October 8-21, 1984:5.
11. PI Perspective. April 1988:7.
12. Rhame FS, Maki DG. The case for wider use of testing for HIV infection. N Engl J Med. 1989;320:1248-1254.
13. Scott GB, Hutto C, Makuch RW, et al. Survival in children with perinatally acquired human immunodeficiency virus type 1 infection. N Engl J Med. 1989;321:1791-1796.
14. Institute of Medicine. HIV Screening of Pregnant Women and Newborns. Washington, DC: National Academy Press; 1991:27.
15. Report of a Consensus Workshop. Early diagnosis of HIV infection in infants, Sienna, Italy, January 17-18, 1992. J Acquir Immune Defic Syndr Hum Retrovirol. 1992;5:1169-1178.
16. Working Group on PCP Prophylaxis in Children. Guidelines for prophylaxis against Pneumocystis carinii pneumonia for children infected with human immunodeficiency virus. MMWR Morb Mortal Wkly Rep. 1991;40(RR-2):1-13.
17. Heagerty MC, Abrams EJ. Caring for HIV-infected women and children [editorial]. N Engl J Med. 1992;326:887-888.
18. Riley J. A bid to disclose infant HIV tests. New York Newsday. May 26, 1993:6.

19. Riley J. HIV-test bill killed. New York Newsday. June 16, 1993:20.

20. It's OK to tell: parents should know HIV results. New York Newsday. May 27, 1993:64.

21. Navarro M. Testing newborns for AIDS virus raises issue of mother's privacy. New York Times. August 8, 1993:1.

22. AIDS babies pay the price. New York Times. August 13, 1993:A26.

23. Not Available. New York Governor's Program, Bill No. 123; 1996.

24. Bateman DA, Cooper A, Abrams EJ. Newborn human immunodeficiency virus testing in New York: a legislative quandary. Arch Pediatr Adolesc Med. 1995;149:581-582.

25. Connor EM, Sperling RS, Gelber R, et al. Reduction of maternal-infant transmission of human immunodeficiency virus type 1 with zidovudine treatment: Pediatric AIDS Clinical Trials Group Protocol 076 Study Group. N Engl J Med. 1994;331:1173-1180.

26. Rovner J. US specialists object to AMA's call for mandatory HIV testing [news]. Lancet. 1996;348:330.

27. Segel AI. Physicians' attitudes towards human immunodeficiency virus testing in pregnancy. Am J Obstet Gynecol. 1996;174:1750-1754.

28. Minkoff H, Willoughby A. Pediatric HIV disease, zidovudine in pregnancy, and unblinding heelstick surveys: reframing the debate on prenatal HIV testing. JAMA. 1995;274:1165-1168.

29. Carusi D, Learman LA, Posner SF. Human immunodeficiency virus test refusal in pregnancy: a challenge to voluntary testing. Obstet Gynecol. 1998;91:540-545.

30. Institute of Medicine. Reducing the Odds: Preventing Perinatal Transmission of HIV in the United States. Washington, DC: National Academy Press; 1998.

31. Shelton DL. Delegates push mandatory HIV testing for pregnant women: American Medical Association House of Delegates vote: annual meeting news. American Medical News. 1996;31:1.

32. Joseph SC. Not Available. Remarks presented at: V International Conference on AIDS; June 4-9, 1989; Montreal, Quebec.

33. Centers for Disease Control and Prevention. Update: public health surveillance for HIV infection: United States, 1989 and 1990. MMWR Morb Mortal Wkly Rep. 1990;39:853-861.

34. Centers for Disease Control and Prevention. HIV/AIDS Surveill Rep. 1997;8(1).

35. Centers for Disease Control and Prevention. Evaluation of HIV case surveillance through the use of non-name unique identifiers: Maryland and Texas, 1994-1996. MMWR Morb Mortal Wkly Rep. 1998;46:1254-1258.

36. Gostin LO, Ward JW, Baker AC. National HIV case reporting for the United States: a defining moment in the history of the epidemic. N Engl J Med. 1997;337:1162-1167.

37. Green J, Arno PS. The "Medicaidization" of AIDS: trends in the financing of HIV-related medical care. JAMA. 1990;264:1261-1266.

38. Deeks SG, Smith M, Holodny M, Kahn JO. HIV-1 protease inhibitors: a review for clinicians. JAMA. 1997;277:145-153.

39. Richman DD. HIV therapeutics. Science. 1996;272:1886-1888.

40. Carton B. New AIDS drug brings hope to Provincetown, but unexpected woes. Wall Street Journal. October 3, 1996:A1.

41. Goldstein A. New treatments put AIDS program in a dilemma. Washington Post. August 15, 1996:A1.

42. National ADAP [AIDS Drug Assistance Program] Monitoring Project. Interim Technical Report. Menlo Park, Calif: Kaiser Family Foundation; March 1998.

43. Casarett DJ, Lantos JD. Have we treated AIDS too well? rationing and the future of AIDS exceptionalism. Ann Intern Med. 1998;128:756-759.

44. Stolberg SG. White House drops plan for Medicaid to cover cost of AIDS drugs for poor. New York Times. December 6, 1997:14.

45. Birmingham K. Clinton's spending on AIDS care goes awry [news]. Nat Med. 1998;4:138. Acquired Immunodeficiency Syndrome; AIDS; AIDS Serodiagnosis; Contact Tracing; Health Services Accessibility; Health Policy; Partner Notification Accession Number: 00000779-199905240-00003

DEBATE QUESTIONS

Once again, we see the conflict between society's health concerns and personal privacy. In this case the societal concern of keeping babies healthy is weighed against a mother's privacy. Here the stakes are quite clear. Which side do you favor? Does this particular situation change your view of privacy rights in general?

Do you see the issue of reporting peoples' names to health registry officials as similar to testing newborns for HIV? Does the question of privacy play a different role in each?

Without saying so explicitly, this article questions whether our principles change with advances in technology. The author lets us know where he stands when he writes, 'Practices uniquely informed by a commitment to privacy rights are increasingly vulnerable to challenge as despair and therapeutic impotence give way to a (perhaps premature) therapeutic trimphalism.' Do you agree that 'commitments to privacy rights' are – or should be – 'vulnerable to challenge'?

Some thoughts on AIDS Exceptionalism and Public Health Sentimentalism[1]

Scott Burris
Assistant Professor of Law, Temple Law School

This article presents another view on the "exceptionalism" doctrine that is discussed above. Has indeed HIV been treated differently? Why are particular measures accepted as applied to some diseases and not as to others? This article represents an approach to the exceptionalism that looks at it from a different angle, arguing against labeling pragmatic approach to disease prevention as an "-ism", that can lead, for example, to the inclusion of obligatory name reporting, that is explained as a trend toward treating all diseases equally. However, even the exceptional history of HIV did not change some traditional approaches to preventable diseases, like improper allocation of available resources to research and treatment, rather than prevention. It is argued that HIV is a typical public health threat to the United States and similarities between AIDS and other leading killer-diseases should be recognized. This will allow better legal protection of people with HIV and will lead to significant shift in public health practice.

IDS, how is it different? How the same? What a rich vein of inquiry, running beneath so many different terrains. 'For the social scientist,' Charles Rosenberg wrote, epidemics constitute an extraordinary useful sampling device – at once found objects and natural experiments capable of illuminating fundamental patterns of social value and individual practice. Epidemics constitute a transverse section through society, reflecting ... a particular configuration of institutional forms and cultural assumptions.'[2] Any number of people have taken Rosenberg's cue and studied the complex data. Susan Sontag has considered AIDS and its Metaphors.[3] Harlon Dalton mediated upon the meaning of AIDS to African Americans.[4] Fee and Krieger wrote of the effort to construct AIDS in the familiar form of past plagues.[5] Mushenow and colleagues have examined judicial behavior in HIV cases.[6] And the list could go on for pages.

The argument that HIV was being treated exceptionally appeared rather early in the epidemic as an instrument of public health policies. Alvin Novick writes:

> The view that AIDS advocates had a gay agenda that was in serious conflict with a proper public health agenda permeated the policy decisions of the Reagan years and was often addressed, directly and obliquely, by Patrick Buchanan and Gary Bauer, both of whom had significant staff positions in the Reagan White House. The concept that federal health policy ... ought to include, or to be directed, at members of groups who were traditionally ostracized and stigmatised, who had already proved to be particularly vulnerable to HIV infection, was anathema to members of the Reagan administration. And so they cast the battle as gay rights versus public health, an articulation now easily recognizable as radically conservative.[7]

Largely serving the needs of rhetoric, this brand of 'exceptionalism' is not an account of HIV and its many forms of meaning and being, but an '-ism,' an enemy ideology which systematically derives a public health policy against HIV from the premise that the disease is essentially different from any other. This is a convenient rhetorical device for advocates of a return to a public health 'tradition,' inasmuch as the premise is so patently untenable, and the conclusion that policy must surely change follows easily. One hopes that Pat Buchanan speaks for a minority of the uninformed, but the belief that HIV has been treated 'differently,' and for purely political reasons, is widely and sincerely held. But has it been? What are the chief elements of this exceptionalism, and how well do they withstand serious scrutiny?

An argument that HIV has been treated differently requires a set of disease that have been treated 'the same.' There must be a norm for there to be a deviance. Bayer's history runs like this:

> It is necessary to recall that conventional approaches to public health threats were typically codified in the latter part of the 19th or the early part of the 20th century. Even when public health laws were revised in subsequent decades, they tended to reflect the imprint of their genesis. They provided a warrant for mandating compulsory examination and screening, breaching the confidentiality of the clinical relationship by reporting public health registries the names of those with diagnoses of 'dangerous diseases,' imposing treatment, and in the most extreme cases, confining persons through the power of quarantine.[8]

This account in indisputable, but on its face it is a statement about law, not practice, and so as a description of history it verges on the tautological. It captures a common sense of the past among some proponents of a 'traditional' HIV policy, but this sort of memory is too short and happy, failing to recall that virtually all these supposedly well accepted measures were at one time or another vigorously disputed. This sort of memory is too fuzzy, supposing that these measures were accepted as Platonic ideals, rather than as applied in particular context to particular diseases. And thus, this sort of memory fails to reach the most important question for public health policy: why are particular measures accepted as applied to some diseases and not as to others?[9]

The answer to this question resides in considering the complex interaction between ideas about disease, disease control, and the proper role of the state. The common practices of health agencies through most of this century reflected a certain 'technology' of disease control – by which I mean a set of measures and an understanding of about how, when, and to whom to apply them – and a social attitude towards that technology and its deployment by the state. Both the technology and social attitudes about its use were rooted in the revolution in biology (and the social status of medicine), entailed in the discovery of specific microbial causes of disease. The success of the germ theory over the last years of the nineteenth century was breathtaking. W.T. Sedgewick, a Massachusetts biologist and public health worker, put it this way: 'before 1880 we knew nothing; after 1890 we knew it all.'[10] The ability to develop vaccines, diagnostic tests, and effective treatments or cures were factors in a general view that 'also provided a rationale for public health officials to disengage themselves from commitments to moral and social reform' that had animated the public health program of the nineteenth century sanitarians. The job of public health on this view was to find patients, and to make sure they got the necessary treatment.[11]

This approach to public health seemed to work. One by one, diseases like tuberculosis, syphilis, polio, diphtheria, and measles were 'conquered' by wonder drugs or vaccines. Smallpox was actually eradicated. So successful was this medical strategy, which was actually implemented more by doctors in the private health care system than public health care workers, that the various health laws authorizing compulsory testing, treatment, or isolation were almost never actually applied.[12] By the1970s, funding for venereal disease and TB control began to decline. Many states repealed pre-marital screening statues as no longer necessary.

Given the frequency of their use, and their deep roots in a medicalized approach to public health, the acceptance of a set of mea-

sures for measles and tuberculosis and hepatitis is far more contin-
gent than public health sentimentalists suggest. Acquiescence to
inaction is hardly acceptance, particularly given the resistance that
often arose when traditional measures were applied.[13] In a larger
sense, the argument that measures like screening and disease
reporting have been accepted implies that the polity (or at least the
targets of the measures) analyze health measures abstractly. The
fact that couples took gonorrhea tests as part of getting a marriage
license, or later allowed their newborns to be tested for PKU, does
not constitute an acceptance of screening as a technology to be
applied to any other condition; just as it is not illogical for people
who do not actively oppose the reporting of measles to oppose government collection of data about sexual intercourse. As a general
matter, public health controversies have little to do with the technical attributes of the measure at issue, but rather turn on more
complex questions of culture, class, and power.

The sentimental account of twentieth century public health
plays on a sprightly theme of historical progress. If one were indel-
icate enough to mention that quarantine was vigorously opposed by
anticontagionist doctors (and laypeople whose livelihood depend-
ed on unfettered commercial trade) throughout the late eighteenth
and nineteenth centuries,[14] or that disease reporting was actively or
passively opposed by physicians throughout the nineteenth century,[15] the response would undoubtedly be that 'we've put that all
behind us.' Once a measure has won its place in the public health
armamentarium, all disputes are forgiven and forgotten. But again,
this is too convenient. The technology of public health has surely
undergone refinement. We can college and analyze information
much better than we could in 1893, but the technology is only part
of the sort of measure may be accepted for one disease but not necessarily for another. Thus, smallpox vaccination did not automati-
cally win public acceptance because it was an improvement over
variolation, any more than the general acceptance of partner notification for venereal disease control compelled its acceptance as
applied to HIV. The same or better measure, even as applied to the

same disease, may have a very different meaning from one time or community to another, and the differing social constructions of different diseases may be far more powerful in shaping the acceptance of a measure than its abstract attributes or its history as applied to other conditions. The use of public education as a weapon against venereal disease in the past hundred years is a case in point.[16]

The notion of progress, when applied to legal doctrine, can also give a deceptive veneer or coherence to the rather disorganized legal treatment of HIV issues in state and federal agencies, courts and legislatures. Some states require HIV reporting, some do not. Some require testing of rape suspects, some virtually ban it.[17] On court allows discrimination against a firefighter with HIV, another condemns it.[18] One finds that firing a nurse with HIV was discrimination, another the appropriate exercise of supervisory authority.[19] Legislation and adjudication reflect local passions and an uneven diffusion of or interest in information about HIV and its control. The idea that early HIV policy was systematically shaped by an ideology of exceptionalism conveniently allows the sentimentalists to declare, based on the adoption of a few screening statutes here and some HIV reporting there, that a pattern of exceptionalism is being replaced by a trend toward 'same-ism.'

Finally, exceptionalism allows the complexity of HIV policy to be reduced to a bilateral conflict between gay men and civil libertarians, and traditionalists. Politics and rights are opposed to public health and the general welfare. The whole enterprise is case as a zero-sum game, so that the declared trend towards more 'traditional' policies at once supports and is supported by the claim that the influence of the original advocates of exceptionalism has begun to wane.[20] Ron Bayer takes this interest group model one step further, suggesting that the steadily increasing proportion of darker and poorer people in the HIV-infected population is the epidemiological equivalent of gerrymandering: 'Not only do black and Hispanic drug users lack the capacity to influence policy in the way that homosexual men have done, but also those who speak on their behalf often lack the singular commitment to privacy and consent that so characterized the posture of gay organizations.'[21]

It has been my experience that gay and civil liberties organizations has had a certain amount of influence that has neither waxed nor waned in any dramatic way and that rights claims, both in politics and in litigation, are normally a lawyer's way of talking about bad health policy, rather than an assertion that public health must be subordinated to individual autonomy.[22] 'Privacy and consent' are also ways of discussing inclusion and social safety, and in health disputes they have often been impossible to disentangle from legal and practical concerns about discrimination. Nothing leads me to believe that advocates for Black or Latin people with HIV are not very concerned about these issues, even if they frame them in terms of empowerment or a fairer use of social resources.

The prime question the sentimentalist's account begs, however, is, why have public health agencies listened to, much less negotiated with, people with HIV? The answer, of course, is not that the Lambda Legal Defense Fund and the ACLU are politically powerful enough to veto any measure they oppose – the claim is belied by the sheer number of terrible HIV policies and statutes enacted across the county. Nor is it because civil rights lawyers can credibly threaten to get undesirable HIV laws overturned after passage, because here the record is one of virtually total failure.[23] The reason that public health policy makers 'had no alternative but to negotiate the course of AIDS policy with representatives of a well-organized gay community and their allies,'[24] and that they will heed the less well-organized voices of drug users, is that health measures that inspire serious resistance among their objects are health measures that will not work. Public health agencies possess the authority, but not really the power, to coerce.[25] Consider, for example, Illinois's premarital HIV-testing statute, a 'traditional' measure miraculously enacted over the objection of the ACLU, and rendered a nullity by the widespread willingness among the marrying kind to take their nuptials elsewhere.[26] Developments in public health practices do not reflect the triumph of one ideology over another, but the continued working of an adaptive process of social negotiation.

Nevertheless, in some important ways, neglected in the sentimental story of exceptionalism, HIV has not challenged the traditionalists' account of public health. For example, most of the money (and most of the advocacy) related to AIDS goes into medical research and treatment. Prevention, given lip service as the only way to stop the epidemic, remains a stepchild of medicine. To the degree the response to AIDS has challenged the medically-centered view of health, however, the challenge is not just to particular measures, but also to the cultural and technological assumptions whose imprint they bear, and indeed the challenge is not raised by HIV advocates alone. As Bayer notes, a public health strategy based on delivering a medical solution to a biological problem has far less force when applied to a behaviourally transmitted disease for which there is no cure,[27] an inconvenience that also makes screening and partner notification less apt. But even were there are cure or vaccine, it would not follow that a traditional strategy would be in order.

Demographic research over the past thirty years has undermined the claim that medical measures were responsible or the dramatic decline of communicable disease since the eighteenth century.[28] Experience with venereal disease and tuberculosis has driven home the point that even the best magic bullets cannot penetrate social barriers to their delivery.[29] Commentators have recognized and wrestled with the frequent disjunction between medical measures promoting individual health and efforts to promote the health of the population as a whole.[30] For many, the future of public health lies less in getting medicine to the sick than in changing the social and physical environments to produce fewer sick people.[31] Instead of concentrating on the delivery of medical interventions, 'Public Health, itself a broad social movement, must in turn generate a succession of specific social movements to deter addictions such as cigarette smoking to shift cultural predilections from unhealthy to healthy foods, or to alter the intimacies of gender scripts that promote the sexual transmission of disease.'[32] For anyone who thinks this way, the tradition that produced a public health strategy focusing on the identification, control and medical treatment of sick individuals is questionable not just as applied to HIV, but also to the diseases against which it was supposedly traditionally applied.

AIDS AS A TYPICAL AMERICAN PUBLIC HEALTH THREAT

HIV, like all diseases, interacts with its environment in a way that reflects the peculiarities of both the virus and the community in which it exists. It is, in other words, unique but not exceptional. For all its uniqueness, however, it is important to see that HIV has much in common with other leading health threats in the United States. Rather than regarding HIV as a throwback to the communicable diseases of the past, we can profitably think of it in the company of other chronic, behaviourally linked threats of affluence – overnutrition, substance abuse, environmentally caused harms.[33]

Public health has been dominated in this century by doctors, by people who tended to think of illness and health in individualistic, biological terms. There is an alternative view, one that understands health as an attribute of communities in social and physical environments. On this view ill health is a complex phenomenon dependent on an interaction of social, biological, genetic, and psychological factors. Improvements in the populations healthful changes in the social and physical environment.[34]

Applying this alternative, ecological perspective, McGinnis and Foege have recently identified the leading nongenetic causes of death in the United States.[35] Their classification system looks past immediate causes of death, based on clinical criteria, to the root causes of ill-health in the social and physical environment. They found that the leading killers in the U.S. today are tobacco (400,000 annual deaths), diet and activity patterns (300,000), and alcohol (100,000). HIV disease was attributed to primarily two causes, sexual behavior (which killed 30,000 people, including most of the 25,000 annual HIV deaths), and illegal drug use (20,000 total, including approximately 9,000 from HIV).

Seen in this light, HIV seems much less exceptional than when we think of it as a sudden viral invader, a throwback to the bubonic plague. It is one of a number of causes of death, like cancer or stroke or heart attack, which medical care alone can do relatively little to prevent or cure, and which can itself be attributed to culturally determined patterns of behavior. That HIV is lethal and incurable makes it like, not unlike, the other leading sources of mortality in America. The focus on behavior change as a primary means of reducing the toll of HIV is likewise unexceptional. Once we accept that ill-health is caused as much by the social and physical environment as by particular microbes or mutations, it follows that reducing ill-health depends heavily on 'social learning' strategies, interventions that aim to change the values, preferences, and behavior of the population.[36]

Disputes between the ecological and medical models of disease are quite common today, at all levels from methodology to the competition for funding. Surgeon General Elders, for example, has made a point of exposing the statistic that only three percent of the money spent on 'health' care goes to preventive measures.[37] There is a debate about the success of particular interventions, like blood pressure screening and treatment, in reducing particular conditions, and about how to measure their success.[38] In research that finds a link between political empowerment and health, the imperative for social change over medical treatment becomes overwhelming.[39] Insofar as the twentieth century public health tradition to which Bayer refers takes a more individualistic, medical view of disease, all the leading modern killers challenge that tradition.

This view of disease and health implies a role for government in shaping of healthier behavior along the full spectrum of social activity. Publically-funded HIV education has provoked strong reactions among people who think that it endorses (homo)sexuality or drug use,[40] but this is not really so different a sort of objection than the claim that measures against smoking infringe upon individual choice, or that limits on violent television would be an impermissible intrusion into freedom to offer or receive ideas. Just as nineteenth century sanitary measures required unfamiliar government meddling with property rights, confronting the problem of unhealthy behavior infringes upon the presently privileged realms of 'privacy' and 'speech.'[41] Perhaps even more unsettling than that, the prospect of the government purposefully manipulating our personal behavior offends the notion that we are autonomous beings making free choices in a marketplace of lifestyles (and, still, occasionally, an idea).[42]

There are good reasons to continue to propose and debate measures to change social values and behavior in a healthy way. My own view is that this sort of governmental manipulation of our desires is a proper use of collective power in a culture where commercial manipulation of individual desires is a billion dollar business. But whether we are talking about AIDS, smoking or double cheeseburgers, the same sorts of issues arise. Here, too, HIV is unexceptional.

DEBATE QUESTIONS

With this article, we have an author who responds *directly* to another article. Burris's main problem with Bayer's argument was the way Bayer framed the issue. For Burris, the issue is not simply 'getting rid of the rights talk and getting back to science.' Do you agree with him?

Burris argues that the public health issue is not a 'zero sum game.' How does he understand Bayer to be framing this issue? Do you agree with Burris or Bayer?

Against the view of public health being a zero sum game, Burris argues for health to be understood 'as an attribute of communities in social and physical environments.' How does this view of public health shift the debate? Do you agree that this is a good way to view public health?

NOTES

[1] Taken from "'AIDS Exceptionalism' and the Law" The John Marshall Law Review 27 pp. 254-264. Used with permission.

[2] Charles E. Rosenberg, "What is an Epidemic? AIDS in Historical Perspective," *Daedalus*, Spring 1989, at 1,2.

[3] Susan Sontag, *AIDS and Its Metaphors* (1988).

[4] Harlon L. Dalton, "AIDS in Blackface," *Daedalus*, Summer 1989m at 205.

[5] Elizabeth Fee and Nancy Krieger, "Thinking and Rethinking AIDS Implications for Health Policy," 23 Int'l J. Health Services 323 (1993).

[6] Michael C. Mushenow et al., "Court Management of AIDS Disputes: A Sociolegal Analysis," 16 L. & Soc. Inquiry 737 (1991).

[7] Alvin Novick, "Judgemental Words and Public Policy," 8 AIDS & Pub Pol'y J. 105, 105 (1993).

[8] Ronald Bayer, "Public Health Policy and the AIDS Epidemic: An End to HIV Exceptionalism?" 324 New England J. Med. 1500 (1991)

[9] Consider Rothman's explanation for the acceptance of coercive measures against tuberculosis carriers early in this century: "Almost no one protested the departments' power to incarcerate persons with tuberculosis, particularly as it became evident that they would exercise their authority almost exclusively against the vagrant and the uneducated immigrant.' Sheila M. Rothman "Seek and Hide: Public Health Departments and Persons with Tuberculosis, 1890-1940," J.L. Med. & Ethics 292 (1993).

[10] Elizabeth Fee, *Disease and Discovery: A History of the Johns Hopkins School of Hygiene and Public Health 1916-1939* (1987).

[11] See Paul Starr, *The Social Transformations of American Medicine: The Rise of a Sovereign Profession and the Making of a Vast Industry* 180-197 (1982).

[12] Bayer, supra note 135, at 1500.

[13] Rothman writes:

To review the history of policy towards tuberculosis in the period 1890-1940 is to find not department of health hegemony over the sick but protracted wars between officials and those with the disease. Regulations which gave health officials authority over persons with tuberculosis also led to a game of seek and hide. Health officials tried to identify, track and isolate patients. Patients subverted the rules or absconded.

Rothman, supra note 136, at 294.

[14] See, e.g. John Duffy, A *History of Public Health in New York City, 1625-1866*, at 134 (1968). For a legal history of quarantine, see Wendy Parmet, *AIDS and Quarantine: The Revival of an Archaic Doctrine*, 14 Hofstra L. Rev. 53 (1985).

[15] See, e.g., Daniel M. Fox, "Social Policy and City Politics: Tuberculosis Reporting in New York 1889-1900," 49 Bull. Hist. Med. 19 (1975). Today, we continue to see major disputes about government data collection. One of the more important Supreme Court cases on privacy, *Whalen v. Roe*, 429 U.S. 589 (1977), concerned the reporting by pharmacists of certain drug prescriptions. For many years, there has been debate (and delay) over governmental efforts to collect data on America's sexual practices, which is nothing more than

behavioural risk factor surveillance.

[16] See generally, Allan M. Brandt, *No Magic Bullet: A Social History of Venereal Disease in the United States Since 1880* (expanded ed. 1987)

[17] Scott Burris, "Testing, Disclosure and the Right to Privacy," in *AIDS Law Today: A New Guide for the Public* 115 (Scott Burris et al. eds., 1993)

[18] Compare *Anonymous Fireman v. City of Willoughby*, 779 F. Supp. 402 (N.D. Ohio 1991) with *Doe v. District of Columbia*, 796 F. Supp. 559 (D.D.C. 1992)

[19] Compare *Leckelt v. Board of Comm'rs of Hosp. Dist. No. 1*, 909 F. 2d 820 (5ᵗʰ Cir. 1990) (private action under 504 of the Rehabilitation Act) with Letter from Davis A. Sanders, Regional Manager, Office for Civil Rights, Regional Office VI, Department of Health and Human Services, to R. James Kellog, Counsel for Kevin Leckelt (Dec. 13, 1989) (on file in Re Terrebone General Medical Center, OCR Docket No. 06-87-2001) [hereinafter HHS Letter] (same complainant's administrative claim against employer).

[20] Bayer, supra note 135, at 1502.

[21] Id. at 1503.

[22] See Scott Burris, "Rationality Review and the Politics of Public Health," 35 Vill. L. Rev. 993 (1989); Scott Burris "Fear Itself: AIDS, Herpes and Public Health Decisions," 3 Yale L. & Pol'y Rev. 479 (1985).

[23] See generally *AIDS Law Today: A New Guide for the Public*, supra note 144 (discussing trends in litigation and legislation). The exception that proves the rule was Utah's ban on marriage by an HIV-positive person. Even the state's attorney general refused to defend its constitutionality. See T.E.P. and K.J.C. v. Michael Leavitt, C.A. No. C-93-653A (D. Utah 1993).

[24] Bayer, supra note 135, at 1502

[25] As Starr has said, "authority signifies a potential to use force or persuasion, though paradoxically authority ends when either of these is openly employed." Starr supra note 138, at 9.

[26] Bernard J. Turnock & Chester Kelly, "Mandatory Premarital Testing for Human Immunodeficiency Virus: The Illinois Experience," 261 JAMA 3415 (1989).

[27] Bayer believes that the availability of early treatment is one of the forces leading to the end of exceptionalism. Unfortunately, much of the promise of early treatment apparent at the time Bayer wrote has (perhaps temporarily) dissipated.

[28] See, e.g., Thomas McKeown, *The Rule of Medicine: Dream Mirage, or Nemesis?* (1979); J. McKinlay & S. McKinlay, "The Questionable Contribution of Medical Measures to the Decline in Mortality in the United States," 55 Millband Q. 405 (1977) (arguing that the introduction of specific medical measures and the expansion of medical services are not responsible for most of the modern decline in mortality rates). But see Samuel Preston, "The Changing Relation Between Mortality and Level Economic Development," 29 Population Stud. 231 (1975).

[29] See, e.g., Brant supra note 143; Sigvi Aral & King Holmes, "Sexually Transmitted Diseases in the AIDS Era," Sci. Am., Feb. 1991, at 62.

[30] Geoffrey Rose, "Sick Individuals and Sick Populations," 14 Int'l J. Epidemiology 32 (1985).

[31] See, e.g. Joycelyn Elders, "The Future of U.S. Public Health," 269 JAMA 2293 (1993); see generally J.S. Feinstein, "The Relationship Between Socioeconomic Status and Health: A Review of the Literature," 71 Millbank Q. 279 (1993).

[32] Mervyn Susser, "Health as a Human Right: An Epidemiologist's Perspective on Public Health," 83 Am. J. Pub. Health 418, 423 (1993).

[33] On the various social constructions of AIDS our culture has produced so far, see Fee & Krieger, supra note 132.

[34] Whether or not, for example, there are genetic co-factors for lung cancer, the most significant cause by far is smoking and the social forces that encourage it. Preventing smoking is, thus, more important to public health than treating cancer. This is not to suggest that medical care is not a concern of public health. Rather, the example serves to challenge the notion, so painfully prevalent in the current medical care reform debate, that health care policy is a proxy for public health.

[35] J. Michael McGinnis & William Foege, "Actual Causes of Death in the United States," 270 JAMA 2207 (1993).

[36] On AIDS and social learning, see Rolf Rosenbrock, "AIDS: Questions and Lessons for Public Health," 8 AIDS & Pub. Pol'yJ. 5 (1993).

[37] Elders, supra note 158, at 2293.

[38] See, e.g. Michele Casper et al., "Antihypertensive Treatment and U.S. Trends in Stroke Mortality," 82 Am. J. Pub. Health 1600 (1992); David Jacobs et al., "U.S. Decline in Stroke Mortality: What Does Ecological Analysis Tell Us?" 82 Am. J. Pub. Health 1596 (1992).

[39] Thomas A. LaVeist, "Segregation, Poverty and Empowerment: Health Consequences for African Americans," 71 Millbank Q. 41 (1992). If people are sick, in part, because of social injustice, then perhaps medical care is the opium of the secular masses.

[40] See Scott Burris, "Education to Reduce the Spread of HIV," in *AIDS Law Today: A New Guide for the Public* supra note 144, at 82.

[41] See Sylvia A. Law, "Addiction, Autonomy, and Advertising," 77 *Iowa L. Rev.* 909 (1992) (discussing the general conflict between regulation of tobacco and alcohol advertising and the First Ammendment).

[42] Howard Leichter, *Free to be Foolish: Politics and Health Promotion in the United States and Great Britain* (1991).

Part 4
Sources

This sources section is divided into two parts. The first part gives the results of three different studies that were conducted on harm reduction. This section is called "Examples of Harm Reduction Initiatives." The second part is a collection of international treaties and guidelines. These two sections should assist you in formulating your ideas on drug policy and HIV/AIDS policy.

A. EXAMPLES OF HARM REDUCTION INITIATIVES

Interventions for Injecting Drug Users[1]

Abu Abdul-Quader, Don Des Jarlais,
Anindya Chatterjee, Elizabeth Hirky & Samuel Friedman

HIV PREVENTION INTERVENTIONS THAT ARE CURRENTLY AVAILABLE

In response to the problem of transmission of HIV among IDUs, a variety of prevention interventions have been implemented in different parts of the world. Some of these interventions have been found to be effective in reducing as well as preventing transmission of HIV. A substantial body of empirical and theoretical evidence demonstrates that a reduction in the sharing of injection drug use equipment significantly reduces HIV transmission rates among IDUs. The following discussion presents brief summaries of some of these interventions that have been used with IDUs. Subsequently, some specific interventions implemented in a selected number of developing countries are reviewed.

EDUCATION OF IDUs

One of the interventions that can facilitate risk reduction is education of IDUs to raise their awareness about the risk of contracting HIV through injection drug use. Studies conducted in the United States have shown the positive impact of educational programs targeting IDUs.[2] In contrast, the impact of a lack of basic factual information about HIV/AIDS can be seen in many areas of Southeast Asia where little AIDS education occurred prior to the initial, rapid spread of HIV among IDUs.

INCREASING AVAILABILITY OF CLEAN INJECTION EQUIPMENT

Making available clean needles and syringes has been very controversial in some countries as a way to prevent HIV among IDUs. Clean needles and syringes can be made available to IDUs through needle and syringe exchange programs, pharmacy-based programs, or pharmacy sale of needles and syringes. Secondary outlets, such as health centers, drug dealers, vending machines, and outreach distribution could be used as well. Because of legal restrictions in many countries, it has been very difficult to implement needle exchange programs.

Evaluation of needle exchange programs around the world shows that they have played a significant role in lowering rates of needle-sharing among IDUs[3-6], and have served as referral sources for other health-related services[7]. Needle exchange programs have also been found not to lead to an increase in drug use nor an increase in HIV drug risk behaviors. Furthermore, HIV infection rates in many cities have remained at stable rate after implementation of needle exchange programs.

DECONTAMINATION OF USED NEEDLES, AND SYRINGES.

There are two effective approaches to inactivate HIV injection equipment: heat and chemicals. Continuous boiling in water for 20 minutes is sufficient to inactivate HIV. However, this may not be a practical option for many IDUs. A second alternative is decontamination using a bleach solution. Bleach is strong and available, and it does not harm the injection equipment or the injector.

Bleach distribution programs were first initiated in San Franscisco and later on in other cities in the United States. The use of bleach was generally accepted by IDUs and, in the absence of syringe exchange programs, bleach was used by a large proportion of IDUs where bleach was distributed.

Although bleach is easily available, and accepted by the IDUs, studies in the United States have failed to show any relationship between self-reported use of bleach to disinfect injection equipment and protection from infection with HIV[8,9]. Several other factors may also determine efficacy of bleach in protecting IDUs from HIV infection. First, the drug users may not know how to "properly" use the bleach to disinfect injection equipment. Second, even if the drug users know how to properly use bleach, they may not be using it properly under "field conditions."[10] The chemical strength of bleach varies from country to country, and it is the free-chlorine concentration in such solutions that governs effectiveness against HIV.

PHARMACOLOGICAL TREATMENT OF DRUG ADDICTION

There are now numerous studies that have demonstrated that participation in pharmacological maintenance treatment, such as methadone maintenance, reduces HIV transmission and acquisition. It has been shown, for example, that risk-associated behavior, incidence of new HIV infection. and overall HIV seroprevalence are significantly lower in IDUs undergoing methadone maintenance treatment than among those not being treated.[11]

OUTREACH AS A METHOD OF INTERVENTION

Since the beginning of the AIDS epidemic, outreach has been initiated in the United States and later on in other countries to educate IDUs about HIV infection and to encourage them to engage in HIV risk reduction behaviors.[12-15] The outreach programs have provided HIV/AIDS prevention information-education materials to IDUs, established links with available services such as drug treatment, HIV counseling and testing, medical care, and social services. The programs often provide some means for engaging in risk reduction behaviors, such as clean syringes, bleach for decontaminating used syringes, and condoms for safer sexual behavior. Most of these programs have hired ex-drug users as peer outreach workers. These outreach interventions have been found to be effective in both reaching IDUs who had never been in any drug treatment program and in reducing HIV risk behaviors.

HIV TESTING

The role of HIV testing in prevention is not conclusive. Studies conducted in the United States and other countries have shown that while testing for HIV may have contributed to the prevention of HIV/AIDS among the general population, the effect among IDUs was not conclusive. In order to use testing for prevention purposes, appropriate counseling must accompany testing. In addition, issues such as anonymity and confidentiality are also important.[16,17]

ORGANIZATION OF IDUs

Establishing organizations of IDUs can have a considerable positive impact on communities where individual IDUs are reluctant to identify themselves because of the legal or stigmatizing environment. In some countries, drug users' organizations have been found to be very helpful in the fight against HIV/AIDS. Such an organization can have many benefits.

The drug users' organization can organize provision of services, such as needle and syringe exchange, have a significant community advocacy role, provide advice to health departments, and be a good mine of information for IDUs. It involves users and ex-users and therefore has close relations with the entire IDU community. This is also a good way to mobilize support and enthusiasm. They act as entry points to other active users. While the relationship between drug users' organizations and HIV/AIDS risk reduction among IDUs was not clear, studies conducted in New York indicated that group efforts to shape the norms of IDUs can lead to increased consistent condom use and bleach use and to decreased syringe sharing, injecting at shooting galleries, and other risk behaviors.[18]

SOCIAL NETWORK INTERVENTION

During the last few years, network intervention techniques have been used to promote risk reduction among IDUs. A drug injector is asked to bring in members of his or her network for a series of group sessions. In the sessions they discuss HIV and how they can work together to protect themselves from infection. Underlying this is the theory that the group has norms and bonds within itself. Thus, they will mutually reinforce each other in their efforts to avoid risk behaviors. The expectation is that the participants in the networks are more likely to change their risk behaviors than those who receive only individually focused intervention. Studies conducted in the United States have shown that participants in the network intervention changed a variety of risk behaviors more than did drug injectors who received an individually focused intervention.[19]

EXPERIENCES FROM DEVELOPING COUNTRIES

Most of these interventions have been implemented in developed countries such as the United States, the countries in Western Europe, and Australia. Since the early 1990s HIV prevention interventions have also been implemented in a number of countries in the developing world. In the following pages we discuss a number of interventions implemented in Asia and Latin America.

Asia
The spread of HIV infection in Asia is of particular significance and concern. Across Asia the prevalence of AIDS in general and

among IDUs in particular varies greatly. The transmission pattern in Asia has been particularly identifiable, as infection patterns are closely linked to drug-producing areas (i.e. the Golden Triangle). HIV infection rates have been further heightened by a change from noninjection to injection drug use and economic factors driving the common practice of sharing needles. Responses to the epidemic of HIV among IDUs in Asia have included drug treatment programs, information-education campaigns, and material outreach programs. Additionally, efforts have been made to garner increased political economic support among government and community organizations for prevention interventions such as bleach distribution and needle exchange that explicitly acknowledge (and some argue sanction) the use of illicit drugs.

The following discussion summarizes the state of the epidemic and among IDUs as well as prevention intervention responses made by select countries in Asia

Thailand

Part of Thailand is in the Golden Triangle of Southeast Asia, which has long been a major center for growing opium. Smoking opium had been the traditional method for using narcotics. This was replaced by heroin injection following law enforcement suppression of opium smoking in the 1960s.

The HIV epidemic among IDUs in Thailand in general and Bangkok in particular is notable for both the rapidity with which the virus spread within the local IDU population and for demonstrating that the problems of HIV infection among IDUs occur in developing as well as industrialized countries. HIV seroprevalence among IDUs in Bangkok increased from approximately 2% in the spring of 1988 to over 40% in the autumn of 1988, with an estimated rate of four new HIV infections per 100 person-months at risk.[20] The spread of the virus was not limited to Bangkok only. High rates of infections were also noted among IDUs in other parts of the country, especially in Northern Thailand. In Bangkok, rapid transmission of HIV wag associated with needle sharing amonng large numbers of IDUs, use of needles and syringes kept by drug dealers (who would lend the needles and syringes to different customers), and incarceration.[21] Whether incarceration as a risk factor was a result of actually "sharing" equipment while injecting in prison or whether incarceration led IDUs to form new social networks with other IDUs (with whom they shared injection equipment after being released from prison) has not yet been determined. However, there may be differences in risk behaviors in other parts of the country.

Bangkok does not have prescription requirements or narcotics paraphernalia laws. Sterile injection equipment can be purchased at a reasonably low cost in pharmacies. There are a large number of methadone maintenance treatment facilities in Bangkok. In response to the epidemic, the IDUs in these programs are provided with HIV risk reduction information and education as well as HIV risk reduction counseling. In addition, HIV prevention information and education campaigns also have been initiated by the authorities. Pharmacy availability of sterile injection equipment combined with these efforts have resulted in decreased sharing of injection equipment and subsequent stabilization of HIV seroprevalence at 40% among the IDUs in Bangkok.[22]

In addition to Bangkok, HIV prevention activities also have been implemented in other parts of the country. These have included drug treatment facilities such as methadone maintenance, syringe-needle distribution, and HIV/AIDS risk reduction information and education. A syringe-needle exchange program was initiated in 1992 in Mae Chan District, Chiang Mai Province in Northern Thailand. Initially the program was implemented in three villages serving approximately 45 IDUs. In 1995, in addition to syringe-needle exchange, primary health care centers were set up and the program was extended to a total of nine villages. In 1998, the program was extended to a total of 12 villages. In 1996, the program began disbursing methadone and tincture of opium to heroin users. HIV seroprevalence among IDUs is lower (17%) than the national rate (40%). Incidence rate among the IDUs in program villages is 2.2%, which is lower than the rate in the north (22%).

Vietnam

There are an estimated 185,000 drug users in Vietnam, of which roughly 50,000 are injectors and the remaining 135,000 use noninjectable drugs.[23] The majority of the injectors are concentrated in urban areas. Traditionally, opium has been smoked in the country. Although a recent decline in the availability of heroin has led to a decrease in heroin use, it also has led to an increase in the use of opium, as well as a change from smoking to injecting opium. Drug users inject a solution, called sai, made from opium and other sedatives. As the price of opium for smoking is high, IDUs mix the residues left after smoking with water and then boil this solution for injecting. Sometimes other sedatives that are available in the market are also added

Risks of HIV transmission among the IDUs are very high because of the high frequency of sharing of injection equipment, shooting gallery use, and the absence of risk reduction measures such as cleaning of injection equipment. In most places the injections are usually administered by the person from whom the IDU is buying the drug. For example, drug dealers and shooting gallery owners usually sell the drugs in a ready-to-use form, that is, ready to be injected from their syringe. Thus, the drug seller usually administers the injection.

HIV was first reported in Vietnam in December 1990, and as of December 1996, there were 4891 reported HIV cases in the country.[24] Most (69.3%) of these HIV infections were among IDUs. Initially, the infections were concentrated mostly in the south, especially Ho Chi Minh City; however, within 6 years, the virus has spread to 43 of the 53 provinces in the country, including those in the far north. Injecting drug use is thought to have played a significant role in the spread of the virus.

Given the prevalence and extent of HIV infections among IDUs, a number of HIV/AIDS intervention programs have been initiated targeting IDUs. About 4 years ago, Save the Children Fund (SCF-UK) initiated a peer education program at the Binh Trieu rehabilitation center in Ho Chi Minh City. Later, the program was extended to IDUs in the community as well as commercial sex workers, street children, and men who have sex with men. The program was implemented in cooperation with local authorities and mass organizations such as the Women's Union and the Youth Union. Since 1993, these outreach programs have contacted more than 4500 IDUs in Ho Chi Minh City, providing information-education for risk reduction in different locations throughout the city including shooting galleries and community locations where IDUs congregate.

In 1995 and later in 1996, SCF-UK implemented experimental syringe exchange programs in Ho Chi Minh City that provided sterile syringes and needles to 175 IDUs. Although the programs were discontinued after only a few months of operation, a survey conducted a year later indicated that 70% of the participants continued to practice safer injection behavior. In addition, many of the users also began to inject at home rather than at shooting galleries

In addition, the National AIDS Committee, in collaboration with local AIDS committees, has initiated peer outreach activities targeting high-risk behaviors including injection drug use in 14 provinces in the country and has provided HIV risk reduction information and education. Although these outreach activities in Ho Chi Minh City and in Hanoi have been in operation for some time, their efficacy in changing behaviors, and thus reducing the risk of HIV transmission, has not yet been assessed.

Nonprescription sterile syringes and needles are available in the pharmacies. Additionally, the costs of purchasing syringes and needles are very low. However, because of the illegal nature of drug use and marginalization of drug users, pharmacy purchase of sterile syringes and needles by the drug users has been difficult. A number of attempts have been made so far to provide sterile syringes and needles to IDUs in Hanoi and Ho Chi Minh City as well as other provinces. These attempts to provide syringes and needles to IDUs have not been very successful and in most cases have been discontinued.

As no evaluation was done, the reasons for discontinuation of syringe and needle distribution could not be ascertained. Although syringes and needles have been distributed to IDUs through out-reach in 14 provinces in the country, no data are available to exam-ine the effectiveness of the outreach as well as the impact of the pro-gram. In addition, the limited information that is available indicates the return rate of used injection equipment was very low (less than 20%). That means that only 20% of the syringes and needles dis-tributed to IDUs were returned by them to exchange for new ones.

In September 1995, the WHO Global Program on AIDS (GPA), in collaboration with the National AIDS Bureau in Vietnam, funded and initiated an intervention project for preven-tion of HIV/AIDS among IDUs that was initiated in Hanoi and Ho Chi Minh City. This is an intervention research study with a pre- and postintervention cross-sectional design.[25] It involves the implementation of intervention activities and an evaluation of their feasibility, efficacy, and impact. The activities include infor-mation dissemination, provision of educational materials, and dis-tribution of sterile syringes and needles on a limited scale, as well as toting and evaluation of the intervention.

The project recruited and trained ex-users as outreach workers to provide HIV/AIDS risk reduction information, condoms, and sterile syringes to IDUs in the community. Distribution of syringes, however, was initiated only after gaining support from community leaders, local law enforcement officials, and health care providers. One of the most important aspects of this program was gaining sup-port from the community and establishing HIV/AIDS as an impor-tant public health problem. The community support was obtained through a series of workshops and seminars attended by communi-ty leaders. With respect to the IDUs, outreach workers initially pro-vided risk reduction information and developed rapport with them before providing syringes.

Preliminary data indicate that the IDUs and the community, including law enforcement authorities, have all been supportive of the syringe-needle exchange program. Data also indicate that the program has been successful in reaching and distributing clean syringes and needles to a large number of IDUs. In Hanoi and Ho

Chi Minh City, the number of IDUs reached by outreach workers doubled within 3 months.[26] Preliminary analyses of follow-up data show initiation of risk reduction by the drug users.

India

Since the late 1980s, the northeastern states of India (Manipur, Nagaland, and Mizoram) have witnessed a tremendous increase in injecting drug use and a subsequent increase in HIV infection among IDUs. Injecting drug use has also been reported in other large cities in the country such as Madras, Calcutta and Delhi, where the drug users have switched from smoking or chasing heroin (beating it in aluminum foil and inhaling it) to injecting synthetic analgesics such as buprenorphine.[27-29]

There is a wide difference in HIV seroprevalence rates among IDUs in India. In Manipur HIV among IDUs is the highest at about 70%. Nagaland has a rate of 50% seroprevalence. A 10% prevalence rate has been reported among IDUs in Mizoram.[30] According to a number of studies, HIV prevalence rates among IDUs in Madras vary between 15 and 20%.[31] In Calcutta, about 1% of IDUs has been found to be infected with HIV.[32] Responses to the epidemic have varied, depending on the extent of the problem as well as the availability of resources and support from the authorities and the larger community. Since the late 1980s and early 1990s, a variety of intervention programs targeting IDUs have been initiated in different parts of India. In some locations a combination of intervention approaches has been used, while in others only one approach has been advocated.

HIV prevention interventions targeting IDUs have been implemented in Calcutta, Delhi, Madras, Bombay, and a number of towns in the states of Manipur, Nagaland, and Mizoram. Most of these interventions include a combination of street-based outreach by ex-users, distribution of HIV/AIDS information and distribution of risk reduction materials such as bleach for cleaning of injection equipment and condoms for safer sex. In Manipur, the intervention approach has also included outreach to family members and friends of IDUs as well as to community members in an attempt to create a supportive environment for the interventions. Advocacy among law enforcement authorities has also been endeavored. In addition, the outreach workers helped the IDUs in forming a drug users' organization. The organization has been found to be very helpful in reaching those IDUs who have not been contacted by the outreach workers.[33]

In Churachandpur, Manipur, the outreach intervention project has reached 700 IDUs and has provided them with HIV/AIDS prevention information-education. Distribution of educational materials has been associated with increased knowledge among IDUs about the risk of sharing of injection equipment. Further, the use of bleach increased from 31 to 72% within 6 months.[34]

Delhi has a relatively large drug-using population. The majority of the users either smoke heroin or inject buprenorphine. Very few interventions have been initiated targeting IDUs in the city. SHA-RAN, a Delhi-based nongovemment organization (NGO) working for the urban poor, has initiated a substitution program where buprenorphine tablets are being provided to buprenorphine injectors and "chasing" and/or smoking heroin.[27]

Interventions in Madras include outreach in the community, provision of risk reduction information and education, distribution of syringes on a limited scale, and drug treatment services. Preliminary data collected in Madras indicate a decline in sharing of injection equipment as well as a decline in injection of buprenorphine. There also has been a decrease in indirect sharing (e.g., sharing of cooker cotton, water). However, condom use still remains low. In Madras, in addition to outreach intervention, personal network-oriented intervention also has been implemented and has been found to be effective in reducing HIV risk behaviors.

In addition, on a limited basis, syringe-needle exchange programs have been implemented in Manipur, Calcutta, and Madras. Most of these programs have been implemented by local NGOs with limited resources and without much political support. The programs' effectiveness have not yet been appropriately assessed or evaluated.

Nepal

It is estimated that there are about 40,000 drug users in Nepal of which heroin is the predominant drug of choice. About 10% of these drug users are injectors. Other drugs that are being used include benzodiazepine, buprenorphine, and barbiturates. Injecting drug use is a recent phenomenon in Nepal. About half of the injectors of the country are in Kathmandu, the main urban center. Syringes are available from pharmacies, but are expensive relative to income. There are six drug treatment centers in Kathmandu and most of them emphasize detoxification.

HIV was first detected in Nepal in 1988. Initially, HIV prevention efforts in the country focused on providing information and education to different population groups. In 1991, the Life and Lifegiving Society (LALS) of Kathmandu began distributing sterile injecting equipment to IDUs in exchange for contaminated equipment. In addition to syringe exchange, LALS also distributes other risk reduction materials, such as sterile water, bleach, and condoms, and provides education, counseling, and primary health care to drug users. The outreach workers of LALS have been in regular contact with about 750 of the 2000 IDUs in Kathmandu. By the end of 1994, there had been 57,734 exchanges.[35] A multiple cross-sectional design has been used to evaluate the program; randomly selected IDUs were interviewed on a yearly basis. This evaluation indicates that there have been significant changes in self-reported injecting behavior and knowledge of HIV among IDUs in Kathmandu from 1991 to 1994. In 1991, 58% of those interviewed knew about HIV/AIDS. By 1994, all the IDUs interviewed knew about HIV/AIDS. HIV risk perception also increased from 25% in 1991 to 47% in 1994. Average number of injections per month decreased from 24 injections in 1991 to 17 injections in 1994. Average number of times of needle sharing per month decreased from 13 in 1991 to 6 in 1994. The overall HIV seroprevalence did not change significantly (1.6% in 1991 and 0% in 1994) and no new HIV-infected individuals were identified in 1993 or 1994. Although there have been significant changes in drug risk behaviors, changes in sexual behavior have not been apparent.[36] Even though the program has shown relative success in reaching IDUs and initiating risk reduction among them, continuous evaluation is needed to examine the program's efficacy in maintaining risk reduction initiated by the IDUs as well as reducing future infections among IDUs.

A few years ago a methadone maintenance treatment (MMTP) was started in Kathmandu. Baseline assessment data indicate that the majority of IDUs enrolled in this MMTP had knowledge of HIV/AIDS. However, half of them reported engaging in needle sharing. While the outcome of the program in terms of reducing drug use and HIV risk is yet to be evaluated, the program in Nepal supports the feasibility of initiating methadone maintenance treatment in a developing country.

Malaysia

It is estimated that there are about 170,000 drug users in Malaysia. Fifty percent of the users use heroin and about 20% are injecting users. HIV infection among IDUs in Malaysia increased from 0.1% in 1988 to 20% in 1994.[37] There are 21 government-operated drug rehabilitation centers in the country at which drug users usually spend about 16 months for first-time treatment. The relapse rate is quite high at 70%, and people who relapse after initial drug treatment usually enter treatment again for approximately another 24 months. Additionally, there are 16 half-way houses run by the government. There are no syringe-needle exchange programs, as the present policies do not allow distribution of sterile injection equipment to IDUs and anyone known to use drugs or aid others in using drugs can be prosecuted.

Although a national AIDS program does exist as part of the Ministry of Health's Division of Disease Control, most of the HIV/AIDS prevention activities to date have been initiated by NGOs. The government allocates funds through its NGO AIDS council to implement these HIV/AIDS activities.

Among different NGOs involved in HIV/AIDS prevention

activities, the IKHLAS project of Pink Triangle has implemented HIV/AIDS risk reduction activities targeting IDUs in Kualalampur. The project operates a drop-in center for drug users and conducts outreach in the community. The drop-in center is open 5 days a week and is where drug users can get medical attention, food, and a place to take a shower and rest. As part of its outreach activities, IDUs in the streets are provided with HIV/AIDS risk reduction information and education and bleach for decontamination of injection equipment.

Evaluation of the program has identified difficulties encountered by IDUs when using bleach under field conditions. However, patterns of consumption among many of the users have been stabilized and many have switched to noninjecting drug use.[38] The relative success of the IKHLAS project has been attributed to the nonjudgmental nature of the program and for creating a 'homelike' safe space for drug users where their voices are heard and where they are treated with respect and importance.[38] In addition to providing HIV/AIDS risk reduction information and education, IKHLAS project also makes referrals to social and health service providers.

Pengasih, an NGO run by former drug users and people with HIV, conducts outreach to drug users on the streets of Kualalampur. While they focus mainly on getting people off drugs, they also provide HIV/AIDS risk reduction information and education and provide social support to other former users and people with HIV. The program has yet to be formally evaluated to assess its efficacy and impact.

Myanmar

Myanmar is one of the countries in Asia that has experienced very rapid spread of HIV among drug injectors. The HIV epidemic in Myanmar began in 1988 with the infection of a large number IDUs; in 1993, the seroprevalence rates among IDUs varied from about 27% in Taunggyi to 95% in Myitkyeena.[39]

It is estimated that there are about 20,000 IDUs in Myanmar. There are major drug treatment centers with a combined daily bed capacity of about 220 to 245 and a yearly capacity of about 2000 to

2200. There are six smaller-scale treatment centers with a combined bed capacity of 125. There are also eight drug rehabilitation centers.[40]

Although the National AIDS Committee, established in 1989, coordinates AIDS prevention and control activities in the country, very few specific interventions have been implemented targeting IDUs. The drug treatment centers and the rehabilitation centers provide information, education, and counseling about HIV and AIDS. Interventions targeting IDUs, however, are limited to the provision of HIV risk reduction information and education. There are no syringe-needle exchange programs.

China

In mainland China, HIV was first detected in 1985. In October 1989, about 100 HIV infections were reported among drug users in treatment in a drug detoxification center in Ruili County, Yunnan Province, southwest China. A study conducted in 1990 in one of the villages in the Yunnan Province found 43% ($N = 182$) of the drug users (both IDU and non-IDU) to be HIV positive. Among the IDUs ($N = 64$), 80% were HIV positive.[41] Another study conducted in the Yunnan Province showed that HIV seroprevalence among the spouses of drug users increased from 3% in 1992 to 10% in 1995.[42]

While the national government has initiated an educational campaign for prevention and control of HIV/AIDS, so far no syringe-needle exchange program has been implemented. A community-based drug abuse prevention program initiated in the southwest focuses more on detoxification and abstinence from drug abuse than on HIV prevention. However, HIV/AIDS risk reduction information and education are also provided. The efficacy of the program in terms of HIV prevention has yet to be evaluated.

Latin America

HIV infection in Latin America initially has been attributed primarily to sexual transmission. However, in a number of countries in this region, injecting drug use played and continues to play a significant role in the spread of the virus. Drug injectors have become the second largest HIV transmission category in Argentina and Brazil. A comparison of the intervention efforts among IDUs in Argentina and Brazil highlights the contrast in magnitude and, to some extent, in the quality and appropriateness of intervention efforts among IDU populations. Intervention efforts in Argentina have been limited both in quantity and quality, while efforts in Brazil have been more extensive and somewhat more comprehensive. The following discussion summarizes the response made by each of these countries to the HIV epidemic among IDUs.

Argentina

It is estimated that there are about 30 to 50 thousand IDUs in Argentina, with the majority residing in Buenos Aires. Injection drug use now accounts for about 40% of all AIDS cases in Argentina. One study conducted in Buenos Aires at two drug rehabilitation centers showed that HIV infection increased from 29% in 1987 to 47% in 1990 for one center and from 38% in 1997 to 46% in 1990 for the others.[43] A similar study conducted in the city of Rosario found an increase in HIV prevalence from 28% in 1988 to 40% in 1990.[44] The rapid spread of HIV among IDUs has been facilitated by a lack of appropriate interventions targeting the IDUs. Injection of cocaine has also contributed to the rapid spread of the virus, primarily due to higher injection frequency resulting from the shorter length of cocaine's effects compared to opiates.

Efforts have been made by local NGOs to try to change public opinion to favor increasing the availability of sterile injection equipment as well as developing and implementing needle and syringe exchange programs. However, these efforts have not passed the discussion stage. Thus, therapeutic programs for IDUs continue to stress drug use abstinence.

Brazil

After the United States, Brazil has the largest number of

HIV/AIIDS cases in the Americas. As of December 1995, Brazil reported 76,396 AIDS cases. Bisexual/ homosexual AIDS cases accounted for 80% of all AIDS cases in 1985. This percentage declined to 41% in 1990 and to 26% in 1995. The proportion of AIDS cases due to injecting drug use increased from 1% during 1982-1985 to 22% in 1995.[45]

The increase in HIV/AIDS among IDUs in Brazil from the mid-1980s to 1995 indicates both an increase in high-risk behaviors among IDUs as well as a lack of effective prevention interventions. A study conducted in Rio de Janeiro with IDUs recruited both from the street and from drug treatment centers found 29% of the participants (n = 72) to be HIV positive.[46] Forty-six percent of the subjects, reported injecting more than once a week and 58% reported having injection equipment. Fifty-one percent reported engaging in unprotected sex with a casual partner. A similar study conducted with IDUs in the city of Santos found 62% of the study participants (N=220) to be HIV positive.[47] Those who were HIV positive reported significantly greater frequency of daily drug injections than those who were HIV negative and less drug-related behavior change (i.e., in cleaning and sharing needles), despite HIV/AIDS awareness

In 1996, a comprehensive HIV prevention program was initiated nationally targeting IDUs. The program includes syringe exchange, drug treatment, outreach intervention, and condom distribution for safer sex. Even though prescriptions are not required to purchase syringes the program has generated much controversy, many local law enforcement officials do not support providing sterile injection equipment to people to use for drug injection. However, syringe exchange programs have been initiated in seven locations in five states.[48] The program has yet to be evaluated to measure effectiveness.

The government also has funded a number of local NGOs to implement interventions targeting IDUs. These interventions have focused mainly on outreach activities through which drug users are provided with risk reduction information and education as well as bleach for syringe decontamination.

In 1989, the city government of Santos declared its intention to start a needle exchange program but it generated a heated public debate and the program could not get off the ground. In 1991, the city government agreed to an educational campaign designed to educate IDUs on decontamination of syringes and needles. An outreach intervention with bleach distribution was initiated in 1993. The program also focused on building trust among drug users and providing risk reduction information and education. Data collected in 1991-1992 indicate that while 52% (N = 220) of the IDUs shared syringes, only 9% of those who shared used bleach. To assess the effectiveness of the program, a selected number (n = 104) of IDUs were interviewed to measure changes in behavior. The results show an increase in the use of bleach. However, no significant changes in needle sharing were reported. Efforts were made to start a users group to facilitate risk reduction among IDUs in Santos. However, no formal evaluation was conducted to measure its impact on risk behavior.

Prevention programs targeting drug users also have been initiated in other parts of the country as well. Most of these programs have focused on providing risk reduction information and health education without any specific intervention such as syringe exchange or bleach distribution. In the city of Porto Alegre, IDUs were asked to join the prevention intervention tem to help develop appropriate outreach messages. In addition to the IDUs, relatives of IDUs and professionals in the health and communication fields were part of the team developing and testing the prevention campaign. Using members from the IDU community helped in the development of appropriate messages as well as in reaching the IDUs. The campaign also helped to generate interest in HIV prevention issues in the local community including local government officials, academia, and the local press. In 1995, a syringe-needle exchange program was initiated in the city of Uvador in the state of Bahia. The program so far has reached about 600 cocaine injectors, and at present 500 to 700 syringes are exchanged per month. In addition to syringes, risk reduction information, condoms, and social and health care support and referrals are also provided to IDUs. Although the program is yet to be formally evaluated, preliminary data collected from IDUs indicate a decrease in needle sharing.

NOTES

[1] Taken from *Preventing HIV in Developing Countries, Biomedical and Behavioral Approaches* eds L. Gibney, R. DiClementi, S. Vermund (New York, Kluwer Academic/Plenum Publishers, 1999) pp. 286-306. Used with permission.

[2] Ostrow DG. AIDS prevention through effective education. *Daedalus* 1989; 118:229 –254.

[3] Institute of Health Policy Studies. The public health impact of needle exchange programs in the United States and abroad: summary, conclusions and recommendations. School of Public Health, University of California, San Francisco, 1993.

[4] Hartgers C, Buning EC, van Santen GW, *et al.* The impact of the needle and syringe-exchange programme in Amsterdam on injecting risk behavior. *AIDS* 1989; 3:571 –576.

[5] Stimson GV. Syringe-exchange programmes for injecting drug users – Editorial review. AIDS 1989; 3: 253-260.

[6] Des Jarlais DC, Maynard H. Evaluation of needle exchange program on HIV risk behaviors: Supplemental final report. American Foundation for AIDS Research, New York, 1992.

[7] Dolan KA, Stimson GV, Donoghoe M. Reduction in HIV risk behavior and stable HIV prevalence in syringe - exchange clients and other injectors in England. *Drug Alcohol Rev* 1993; 12:133 – 142.

[8] Vlahov D, Astemborski J, Solomon L, Nelson KE. Field effectiveness of needle disinfecting among injecting drug users. *J Acquir immunodefic Syndrs* 1994; 7:760 – 766.

[9] Titus S, Marmor M, Des Jarlais DC, *et al.* Bleach use and HIV seroconversion among New York City injection drug users. *J Acquir immunodefic Syndrs* 1994; 7:700 – 704.

[10] Gleghorn AA, Doherty MC, Vlahov D, *et al.* Inadequate bleach contact times during syringe cleaning by injection drug-users. *J Acquir immunodefic Syndrs* 1994; 7:762 – 772.

[11] Caplehorn JR, Ross MW. Methadone maintenance and the likelihood of risky needle sharing. *Int J Addict* 1995; 30:685 – 698.

[12] Neaigus A, Sufian M, Friedman SR, et al. Effects of outreach intervention on risk reduction among intravenous drug users. *AIDS Educ Prevent* 1990; 2:253-271.

[13] Centers of Disease Control. Assessment of street outreach for HIV prevention-selected sites, 1991-1993. MMWR 42(45):873, 879-880.

[14] Abdul- Quader AS, Des Jarlais DC, Tross S, et al. Outreach to injecting drug users and female sexual-partners of drug-users on the Lower East Side of New York City. Br J Addict 1992; 87:519-526.

[15] Weibel W, Jimenez A, Johnson W, et al. Positive effect on HIV seroconversion of street outreach intervention with IDU in Chicago: 1988-1992. 9th International Conference on AIDS, Berlin, 1993. Abstract No. WS-C15-2.

[16] Cartter ML, Petersen LR, Savage RB, Donagher J. Providing HIV counseling and testing services in methadone maintenance programs. AIDS 1990; 4 (5):463 – 465.

[17] Higgins DL, Galavotti C, O'Reilly KR, et al. Evidence for the effects of HIV antibody counseling and testing on risk behaviors. JAMA 1991; 266:2419–2429.

[18] Friedman SR, Des Jarlais DC, Neaigus A, et al. Organizing drug injectors against AIDS: Preliminary data on behavioral outcomes. Psychol Addict behav 1992; 6:100 – 106.

[19] Latkin CA, Mandell W, Vlahov D, et al. The long-term outcome of a personal network-oriented HIV prevention intervention for injection drug users: The SAFE study. Am J Commun Psychol 1996; 24: 341–364.

[20] Vanichseni S, Sakuntanaga P. Results of three seroprevalence surveys for HIV and IVDU in Bangkok. Sixth International Conference on AIDS, San Francisco, CA, 1990.

[21] Choopanya K, Vanichseni S, Des Jarlais DC, et al. Risk factors and HIV seropositivity among injecting drug users in Bangkok. AIDS 1991; 5:1509 –1513.

[22] Des Jarlais DC, Choopanya K, Wenston, et al. Risk reduction and stabilization of HIV seroprevalence among drug injectors in New York City and Bangkok, Thailand. In: Rossi GB, Beth-Giraldo E, Chieco- Bianchi L, et al., (Eds.) Science Challenging AIDS. Basel: Karger, 1992; 207 –213.

[23] Government of Socialistic Republic of Vietnam. Vietnam National Drug Abuse Control Plan. Hanoi; 1995.

[24] Vietnam National AIDS Committee. Annual Report. Hanoi; 1996.

[25] Vietnam National AIDS Committee. Harm Reduction for Injecting Drug Users. Hanoi; 1995.

[26] Quan VM, Chung A, Abdul -Quader AS. Feasibility of a syringe –needle exchange program in Vietnam. Substance Use Misuse 1998; 33 (5): 1-14.

[27] SHARAN – Annual Report. New Delhi, 1995.

[28] Kumar S, Daniels D. HIV risk reduction strategies among IDUs in Madras: Assessment research report. Madras, India; 1994.

[29] Stimson GV. The global diffusion of injecting drug use: implications for human immunodeficiency virus infection. Bull Narcotics 1993; 45(1):3-17.

[30] Indian Council of Medical Research. Annual Report. Calcutta, 1995.

[31] Kumar S, Daniels D. Empirical evidence of behavior change. Paper presented at the Indo –US Workshop on Behavioral and Social Research on HIV Prevention. Bombay, 1996.

[32] Panda S, Chatterjee A, Sarkar S, et al. Injection drug use in Calcutta: A

potential focus for an explosive HIV epidemic. *Drug Alcohol Rev* 1997; 16:17 – 23.

[33] Hangzo C, Chatterjee A, Sarkar S, et al. Reaching out beyond the hills: HIV prevention among injecting drug users in Manipur, India. *Addiction* 1997; 92 (7): 813 –820.

[34] Chatterjee A, Hangzo CZ, Abdul- Quader AS, et al. Evidence of effectiveness of street-based peer outreach intervention to change behavior among injecting drug users in Manipur, India. XI International Conference on AIDS, Vancouver, 1996. Abstract No. 4975

[35] Peak A, Rana S, Maharjan SH, et al. Declining risk for HIV among injecting drug users in Kathmandu, Nepal: The impact of a harm reduction programme. AIDS 1995; 9:1067 – 1070.

[36] Shreshtha DM, Shreshtha NM, Gautama K. Methadone treatment programme in Nepal: A one-year experience. *J Nepal Med Assoc* 1995; 33:33 – 46.

[37] AIDSCAP/Family Health International. Harvard School of Public Health, and UNAIDS. The Status and Trends of the Global HIV/AIDS Pandemic Symposium Final Report. Vancouver, 1996.

[38] Palaniappan N. Intervention among multiracial injecting drug users from different cultural and economical backgrounds. XI International Conference on AIDS, Vancouver, 1996. Abstract No. Mo.D. 1949.

[39] Htoon MT, Lwin HH, San KO, et al. HIV/AIDS in Myanmar. AIDS 1994; 8(suppl 2): S105- S109.

[40] Stimson GV. HIV infection and injecting drug use in the Union of Myanmar: Final report to the United Nations Drug Control Programme, Vienna, Austria, 1994.

[41] Xia M, Kreiss JK, Holmes KK. Risk factors of HIV infection among drug users in Yunnan Province, China: Association with intravenous drug use and protective effect of boiling reusable needles and syringes. *AIDS* 1994; 8:1701-1716.

[42] Zheng X, Zhang J, Qu X, et al. The sero-prevalence and incidence rates of HIV infection among IDUs by cohort study from 1992 to 1995 in Ruili and other countries of China. XI International Conference on AIDS, Vancouver; 1996. Abstract No. Tu.C. 2515.

[43] Libonatti O, Lima E, Peruga A, et al. Role of drug injection in the spread of HIV in Argentina and Brazil. *Int J STD AIDS* 1993; 4:135-141.

[44] Fay O, Taborda M, Fernandez A, et al. HIV seroprevalence among different communities in Argentina after four years of surveillance. VII International Conference on AIDS, Florence, Italy; 1991. Abstract No. M.C.3263.

[45] Chequer P, Castilho E, Gomes MRO, et al. Fifteen years of AIDS epidemic in Brazil: Trends over time and perspectives. XI International Conference on AIDS, Vancouver; 1996. Abstract No Mo.C.1439.

[46] Rangel A, Telles P, Bastos F, et al. HIV risk in IDUs in Rio de Janeiro: Psychological Predictors and implications for intervention. XI International Conference on AIDS; Vancouver; 1996. Abstract No. Tu.C.2495.

[47] de Carvalho HB, Mesquita F, Massad E, et al. HIV and infection of similar

transmission patterns in a drug injectors community of Santos, Brazil. *J Acquir Imunne Defic Syndr Hum Retrovirol* 1996; 12(1):84 – 92.

[48] Loures LA, Bittencourt L, Marques F, *et al*. Dealing with a paradox: The national syringe exchange program in Brazil. XI International Conference on AIDS, Vancouver; 1996. Abstract No. We.C.3562.

Syringe Exchanges: A Public Health Response to Problem Drug Use. Discussion[1]

GM Cox, MC Lawless, SP Cassin & TW Geoghegan
The Merchant's Quay Project, Dublin, Ireland

This study has shown that syringe exchange programs can be highly effective as a public health initiative. The changes in reported primary drug use, and frequency of use could be simply ascribed such external market forces as low/non availability of heroin and a greater availability of prescribed drugs such as methadone. Yet the absence of any reported increases in drug use along with the substantial increase in more hygienic injecting practices indicates both the willingness and the capacity of this drug using population to effect change.

While, one of the primary aims of any syringe exchange is, in as far as possible, to eliminate the sharing of used injecting equipment, the results, although positive, highlight a number of issues of concern. In theory, increased availability of injecting equipment should reduce the necessity to share (the circulation theory).[2] The term sharing covers two aspects of joint use of injecting equipment, borrowing and lending, which differ markedly in terms of personal risk.[3]

This study illustrated a significant reduction in both the borrowing and lending of used injecting equipment by respondents at the three-month follow-up intervention. Evidence from international studies support these findings, for example Caslyn et al. (1991) found that the proportion of injectors who share in areas where clean injecting equipment is available is lower (78%) than areas where there is restricted access (98%).[4] Other research has shown lower rates of sharing among syringe exchange attendees when compared with non-attendees[5] and studies comparing baseline measures among syringe exchange attendees with post entry measures have also shown a reduction in sharing.[6]

There is no doubt that the availability of sterile injecting equipment (or lack thereof) impacts on the levels of sharing.[7] This is of particular relevance to the situation in Dublin where syringe availability remains limited.[8] The Merchant's Quay Project is the only voluntary sector syringe exchange and the only five day a week service in Dublin. This lack of access to syringe exchange services at week-ends and evening times, represents a serious deficit in service provision. Service development should include syringe exchanges at local and community level, strategically placed vending machines, mobile syringe exchanges and pharmacy involvement in needle/syringe distribution could address this situation. However, increased availability cannot eliminate all sharing behavior, as environmental, economic, cultural and social factors can result in a situation in which needle sharing takes place.[9]

Despite the positive changes in the lending and borrowing of injecting equipment, minimal changes in the sharing of injecting paraphernalia were reported. This is of concern as research illustrates that the sharing of spoons and filters is likely to be a major cause of the spread of HIV and HCV infection. Although the results of this study suggest that among injecting drug users there is a high level of knowledge and practice to prevent HIV, less importance is given to hepatitis C transmission. It is vital that greater emphasis be placed on disseminating information on HCV transmission as part of a syringe exchange intervention to ensure that injecting drug users perceive the sharing of injecting paraphernalia as potentially risky behavior. To this end, there is a need to target drug users, with a variety of educational and awareness programs similar to those done for HIV in the 1980's and 1990's. Given the high levels of HCV infection among drug users with up to an 80% infection rate reported in Dublin studies,[10] this matter is of serious concern.

The fact that as many as half of the sample reported their initial presentation at the Health Promotion Unit as being their first treatment contact places the role of health promotion within a syringe exchange to the fore in forging earlier contact with the drug using population. To this end, a more proactive approach could be adopted. The provision of outreach services, including syringe exchange, to deal specifically with the 'hard to reach,' such as, injecting drug users who have not maintained contact of have never initiated contact with a syringe exchange, will ensure a more effective public health response.

Changes in sexual behavior, in particular the use of condoms, were less marked than changes in injecting practices. Although there was no significant change in the percentage of clients who reported having had a regular sexual partner, 30% of follow-up clients reporting movement in and out of such a relationship within the time period (n=110). These findings highlight the importance of advising drug users on sexual risk behavior in addition to injecting risk behavior.

Almost all studies have reported low levels of condom use among drug users with little improvement over time.[11] Research studies highlight that harm reduction interventions have tended to focus less on changing the sexual behavior of drug injectors and also suggest that in instances where such interventions are made the outcome is not always effective.[12]

The emphasis placed on needles and syringe sharing has tended to lead to the exclusion of other risk factors.[13] As drug users continue to reduce the individual harms directly associated with drug use, sexual transmission is becoming increasingly important in determining the future dynamics of the HIV epidemic spread.

There remains a significant risk of HIV transmission to the non-injecting partners of drug injectors, in particular women.[14] The limited aspect of interventions on sexual risk behavior is a matter of serious concern. It is vital that a greater emphasis be placed on promoting safer sex practices as an integrated component of syringe exchange services. Encouraging needle exchange users to discuss their sexual practices with a view to adopting safer sexual practices is a highly skilled intervention. Service providers engaged in low threshold and health promotion approaches to harm reduction will need to provide training for staff to ensure that they have the skills and competencies to address the issue of sexual risk behavior more effectively.

Finally, the results of this study illustrate that the possibility of making interventions in the overall health and welfare of clients is significant, given the particular range and level of health complaints reported by attendees. The provision of more traditional medical inputs on site within a syringe exchange could prove invaluable in addressing other primary health concerns such as abscesses, soft tissue damage and other infections in addition to providing screening services for HIV/HCV and vaccinations. This level of medical intervention could offer significant health gain not only for the individual drug user but also in the wider public health context at a societal level.

The origins of drug treatment in Ireland are from a total abstinence background and it is only in more recent years that syringe exchanges have become more widely accepted as a valid component of drug treatment. While progress has been made, syringe exchange programs still represent one of the least socially acceptable faces of drug treatment and have proved difficult to establish at community level in Dublin. The results of this study, supported international research which illustrate that syringe exchanges are an effective public health response to problem drug use. However, the study also highlights a number of deficits in terms of service provision which will have toe be addressed in the Irish context if syringe exchanges are to maximize their potential as public health initiatives.

NOTES

[1] Taken from "Syringe Exchanges: A Public Health Response to Problem Drug Use" Irish Medical Journal 93(5) July-August 2000 pp. 143-146. Used with permission.

[2] Kaplan, E, and R. Heimer. A Circulation Theory of Needle-Exchange. AIDS 1994:8:567-74

[3] Klee, H, Faugier, J, Hayes, C, and J. Morris, Risk Reduction Among Injecting Drug Users. Changes in the Sharing of Injecting Equipment and Condom Use. AIDS Care 1991:3:1:63-73

[4] Caslyn, D. et al. Needle-Use Practices Among Intravenous Drug Users in an Area where Needle Purchase in Legal. AIDS 1991:5:187-93

[5] See Donoghoe, M, Stimson, G, Dolan, K and L Alldritt Changes in HIV Risk Behaviour in Clients in Syringe-Exchange Schemes in England and Scotland. AIDS 1989:3:267-272; Hartgers et al. The Impact of the Needle-Exchange Programs in Amsterdam on Unjecting Risk Behaviour. AIDS. 1989:3571-76; Keene, J, et al Evaluation of Syringe Exchange for HIV Prevention among Injecting Drug Users in Rural and Urban Areas of Wales. Addiction. 1993:868:1063-70.

[6] See Hart et al.. Evaluation of needle-exchange in central London: Behaviour change and Anti-HIV Status Over One Year. AIDS. 1989:3:571-76;Hagan, H, et al. An Interview Study of Participants in the Tacoma. Washington Syringe-Exchange. Addiction, 1994:98:191-202; Saxon, A, Calsyn, D, and R. Jackson. Longitudinal Changes in Injecting Behaviours in a Cohort of Injecting Drug Users. Addiction. 1994:89:1691-97.

[7] Kaplan, E. and R. Heimer. A Circulation Theory of Needle-Exchange. AIDS 1994:8:567-74

[8] Farrel et al External Review of Drug Services for the Eastern Health Board. National Addiction Centre: Institute of Psychiatry, London, 2000.

[9] See Donoghoe, M., Stimson, G., Dolan, K., and L. Alldritt. Changes in HIV Risk Behaviour in Clients in Syringe-Exchange Schemes in England and Scotland. AIDS 1989:3:267-272. Klee et al. The Sharing of Injecting Equipment among Drug Users attending Prescribing Clinics and those using Needle-Exchanges. British Journal of Addiction 1991:86:217-223.

[10] Smyth, R et al. Hepatitis C Infection among Injecting Drug Users Attending the National Drug Treatment Centre. Irish Journal of Medical Science. Oct/Dec. 1995: 267-268.

[11] See Hartgers et al. The Impact of the Needle-Exchange Programmes in Amsterdam on Injecting Risk Behaviour. AIDS. 1989:3:261-265.Rhodes, T. et al. Sexual Behaviour of Drug Injectors in London: Implications for HIV Transmission and HIV Prevention. Addiction. 1994:89:1085-96. Donoghoe, M. Sex, HIV and the Injecting Drug User. British Journal of Addiction. 1992:87:405-16. McKeganey, N. Barnard, M. and H. Watson. HIV Related Risk Behaviour Among a Non-Clinic Sample of Injecting Drug Users. British Journal of Addiction. 1989:84:1481-490.

[12] Donoghoe, M. Sex, HIV and the Injecting Drug User. British Journal of

Addiction. 1992:87:405-16.

[13] Hart, G. Injecting Drug Use, HIV and AIDS in AIDS Care. 1989:1:3:237-245.

[14] Rhodes, T. *et al.* Sexual Behaviour of Drug Injectors in London: Implications for HIV Transmission and HIV Prevention. Addiction. 1994:89:1085-96.

Decline in Self-Reported High-Risk Injection-Related Behaviors Among HIV-Seropositive Participants in the Baltimore Needle Exchange Program[1]

John Vertefeuille, Melissa Ann Marx, Waimar Tun,
Steven Huettner, Steffanie A. Strathdee
& David Vlahov

The major finding of this study is that after enrolling in NEP, HIV seropositive IDUs reduced risky drug injection behaviors that would likely contribute to transmission of their HIV infection to other injectors. Several previously published reports from NEPs in the United States and Europe have indicated that needle exchange can be effective in reducing the transmission of blood-borne pathogens (Des Jarlais *et al.* 1996; Heimer, 1998b; Vlahov and Junge, 1998; Vlahov *et al.*, 1997). This study suggests that NEP may also specifically reinforce positive behavior change in HIV-infected participants. This reduction in risky injection-related behaviors by HIV-seropositive individuals can help decrease the risk of transmission of HIV and other blood-borne pathogens in this population.

Several limitations of this study should be considered. First, the lack of an external comparison group in this study may imply that the observed behavior change was due to factors other than NEP attendence. Second, all NEP participants are self-selected into the NEP. These individuals may well have changed their behavior regardless of NEP enrollment. Third, the reliability of self-reporting is another possible limitation of this study. However, a recently published review determined that, in fact, the inaccuracies associated with socially desirable reporting tend to result in an overreporting, rather than an underreporting of risk behaviors (Darke, 1998). This contradicts the results reported in a recent study of NEP participants that indicated significantly higher self-reports of drug use and HIV risk behavior was seen when audio-computer-assisted self-interviews were used rather than face-to-face interviews (Des Jerlais et al., 1999). This work by Des Jerlais et al. suggests that self-report of sensitive HIV and IDU risk behaviors may be underreported in face-to-face interviews (such as the ones used in this study). However, the same article reports the despite its findings, face-to-face interview data can still be viewed as highly valid and reliable (Des Jerlais et al., 1999). Bias due to self-reporting of risky behaviors, however, should be negligible in the present study, since participants acted as their own control from baseline to 6-month follow up. Recall bias is unlikely to be a source of bias in the present study because most questions refereed to a 2-week period prior to the interview. Finally, an additional limitation to this study is the lack of comprehensive utilization statistics for NEP participants. Utilization patterns could influence the interpretation of the study findings in terms of how the degree of NEP usage is associated with the documented behavior change.

In spite of these limitations, the significant reduction in direct needle sharing that was found among HIV-infected IDUs in this study is encouraging. Significant reductions were noted both in the lending of syringes to others as well as the borrowing of used syringes. The availability of sterile, economically ascertainable needles through needle sharing suggests that this reduction is likely to be associated with NEP participation. Our findings showed an 18.5% decline in lending of used syringes to others and a 12.1%

decline in borrowing syringes over the 6-month period. These find-ings are consistent with the reductions seen in needle sharing among a group of NEP attendees consisting of HIV-seropositive and HIV-seronegative participants (lending to friends decreased by 14.7% and borrowing syringes decreased 13.6% over a 6-month period in a study by Vlahov et al., 1997; see also (Des Jerlais et al., 1996; Hagan et al., 1995). Implications of these findings are that HIV-seropositive NEP participants will be less likely to spread HIV to others through injection drug use. Furthermore, these HIV-infected IDUs are less likely to become infected with blood-borne pathogens because of the reductions in borrowing syringes used by other people. The reduction seen in sharing of injection-related equipment (cookers and cotton) suggest that NEP also promotes reductions of risk sharing of these items. The significant decrease in injection at shooting galleries supports our hypothesis that the use of such high-risk venues declines when reliable sources of syringes and other injection equipment are available. It is worth noting that this would require conscious behavior change on the part of the individual because NEP does not offer a physical setting for injec-tion. The data suggest that there was no increased injection in pub-lic places and that there was a statistically significant decrease in reported injection in abandoned buildings after enrolling in NEP. These results indicate that the presence of needle-exchange does not increase the amount of injection in such areas for HIV-seropositive IDUs, which is consistent with results previously seen among NEP participants as a whole, regardless of HIV status (Vlahov et al., 1997). These data, when taken together, begin to provide insight into the role of needle exchange in IDU behavior change. Finally, the reduction in the number of injections and the significant increase in reported drug treatment participation sug-gests that needle exchange may provide a bridge to treatment for HIV-seropositive IDUs, as has been suggested in other studies (Brooner et al., 1998; Heimer, 1998a).

The results obtained in this study suggest that NEP use can result in reduction of risky injection behaviors among HIV-seropositive participants. The implications of such results are that NEP will serve as an important intervention for curbing the HIV epidemic in this high-risk population. These results are in accord with numerous other studies conducted to evaluate the effectiveness of needle exchange for reducing risky injection practices in the IDU population (Des Jerlais *et al.*, 1996; Hagan *et al.*, 1995; Vlahov *et al.* 1997). Unlike other studies, however, the present report emphasizes that these reductions occur in the HIV-seropositive participants, suggesting that NEP may provide an impetus for behavior change among individuals who have an increased probability of spreading HIV through unsafe injection behaviors.

NOTES

[1] Taken from AIDS and Behavior 2000 pp. 385-7. Used with permission.

B. HUMAN RIGHTS TREATIES AND GUIDELINES

Declaration of Commitment on HIV/AIDS "Global Crisis — Global Action"

1. We, Heads of State and Government and Representatives of States and Governments, assembled at the United Nations, from 25 to 27 June 2001, for the twenty sixth special session of the General Assembly convened in accordance with resolution 55/13, as a matter of urgency, to review and address the problem of HIV/AIDS in all its aspects as well as to secure a global commitment to enhancing coordination and intensification of national, regional and international efforts to combat it in a comprehensive manner;

2. Deeply concerned that the global HIV/AIDS epidemic, through its devastating scale and impact, constitutes a global emergency and one of the most formidable challenges to human life and dignity, as well as to the effective enjoyment of human rights, which undermines social and economic development throughout the world and affects all levels of society — national, community, family and individual;

3. Noting with profound concern, that by the end of the year 2000, 36.1 million people worldwide were living with HIV/AIDS, 90 per cent in developing countries and 75 per cent in sub-Saharan Africa;

4. Noting with grave concern that all people, rich and poor, without distinction of age, gender or race are affected by the HIV/AIDS epidemic, further noting that people in developing countries are the most affected and that women, young adults and children, in particular girls, are the most vulnerable;

5. Concerned also that the continuing spread of HIV/AIDS will

constitute a serious obstacle to the realization of the global development goals we adopted at the Millennium Summit;

6. Recalling and reaffirming our previous commitments on HIV/AIDS made through:

- The United Nations Millennium Declaration of 8 September 2000;

- The Political Declaration and Further Actions and Initiatives to Implement the Commitments made at the World Summit for Social Development of 1 July 2000;

- The Political Declaration and Further Action and Initiatives to Implement the Beijing Declaration and Platform for Action of 10 June 2000;

- Key Actions for the Further Implementation of the Programme of Action of the International Conference on Population and Development of 2 July 1999;

- The regional call for action to fight HIV/AIDS in Asia and the Pacific of 25 April 2001;

- The Abuja Declaration and Framework for Action for the Fight Against HIV/ AIDS, Tuberculosis and other Related Infectious Diseases in Africa, 27 April 2001;

- The Declaration of the Ibero-America Summit of Heads of State of November 2000 in Panama;

- The Caribbean Partnership Against HIV/AIDS, 14 February, 2001;

- The European Union Programme for Action: Accelerated Action on HIV/ AIDS, Malaria and Tuberculosis in the Context of Poverty Reduction of 14 May 2001;

- The Baltic Sea Declaration on HIV/AIDS Prevention of 4 May 2000;

- The Central Asian Declaration on HIV/AIDS of 18 May 2001;

7. Convinced of the need to have an urgent, coordinated and sustained response to the HIV/AIDS epidemic, which will build on the experience and lessons learned over the past 20 years;

8. Noting with grave concern that Africa, in particular sub-Saharan Africa, is currently the worst affected region where HIV/AIDS is considered as a state of emergency, which threatens development, social cohesion, political stability, food security and life expectancy and imposes a devastating economic burden and that the dramatic situation on the continent needs urgent and exceptional national, regional and international action;

9. Welcoming the commitments of African Heads of State or Government, at the Abuja Special Summit in April 2001, particularly their pledge to set a target of allocating at least 15 per cent of their annual national budgets for the improvement of the health sector to help address the HIV/AIDS epidemic; and recognizing that action to reach this target, by those countries whose resources are limited, will need to be complemented by increased international assistance;

10. Recognizing also that other regions are seriously affected and confront similar threats, particularly the Caribbean region, with the second highest rate of HIV infection after sub-Saharan Africa, the Asia-Pacific region where 7.5 million people are already living with HIV/AIDS, the Latin America region with 1.5 million people living with HIV/AIDS, and the Central and Eastern European region with very rapidly rising infection rates; and that the potential exists for a rapid escalation of the epidemic and its impact throughout the world if no specific measures are taken;

11. Recognizing that poverty, underdevelopment and illiteracy are among the principal contributing factors to the spread of HIV/AIDS and noting with grave concern that HIV/AIDS is compounding poverty and is now reversing or impeding development in many countries and should therefore be addressed in an integrated manner;

12. Noting that armed conflicts and natural disasters also exacerbate the spread of the epidemic;

13. Noting further that stigma, silence, discrimination, and denial, as well as lack of confidentiality, undermine prevention, care and treatment efforts and increase the impact of the epidemic on individuals, families, communities and nations and must also be addressed;

14. Stressing that gender equality and the empowerment of women are fundamental elements in the reduction of the vulnerability of women and girls to HIV/AIDS;

15. Recognizing that access to medication in the context of pandemics such as HIV/AIDS is one of the fundamental elements to achieve progressively the full realization of the right of everyone to the enjoyment of the highest attainable standard of physical and mental health;

16. Recognizing that the full realization of human rights and fundamental freedoms for all is an essential element in a global response to the HIV/AIDS pandemic, including in the areas of prevention, care, support and treatment, and that it reduces vulnerability to HIV/AIDS and prevents stigma and related discrimination against people living with or at risk of HIV/AIDS;

17. Acknowledging that prevention of HIV infection must be the mainstay of the national, regional and international response to the epidemic; and that prevention, care, support and treatment for those infected and affected by HIV/AIDS are mutually reinforcing elements of an effective response and must be integrated in a comprehensive approach to combat the epidemic;

18. Recognizing the need to achieve the prevention goals set out in this Declaration in order to stop the spread of the epidemic and acknowledging that all countries must continue to emphasize widespread and effective prevention, including awareness-raising campaigns through education, nutrition, information and health-care services;

19. Recognizing that care, support and treatment can contribute to effective prevention through increased acceptance of voluntary and confidential counselling and testing, and by keeping people living with HIV/AIDS and vulnerable groups in close contact with health-care systems and facilitating their access to information, counselling and preventive supplies;

20. Emphasizing the important role of cultural, family, ethical and religious factors in the prevention of the epidemic, and in treatment, care and support, taking into account the particularities of each country as well as the importance of respecting all human rights and fundamental freedoms;

21. Noting with concern that some negative economic, social, cultural, political, financial and legal factors are hampering awareness, education, prevention, care, treatment and support efforts;

22. Noting the importance of establishing and strengthening human resources and national health and social infrastructures as imperatives for the effective delivery of prevention, treatment, care and support services;

23. Recognizing that effective prevention, care and treatment strategies will require behavioural changes and increased availability of and non-discriminatory access to, inter alia, vaccines, condoms, microbicides, lubricants, sterile injecting equipment, drugs including anti-retroviral therapy, diagnostics and related technologies as well as increased research and development;

24. Recognizing also that the cost availability and affordability of drugs and related technology are significant factors to be reviewed and addressed in all aspects and that there is a need to reduce the cost of these drugs and technologies in close collaboration with the private sector and pharmaceutical companies;

25. Acknowledging that the lack of affordable pharmaceuticals and of feasible supply structures and health systems continue to hinder an effective response to HIV/AIDS in many countries, especially for the poorest people and recalling efforts to make drugs available at low prices for those in need;

26. Welcoming the efforts of countries to promote innovation and the development of domestic industries consistent with international law in order to increase access to medicines to protect the health of their populations; and noting that the impact of international trade agreements on access to or local manufacturing of, essential drugs and on the development of new drugs needs to be further evaluated;

27. Welcoming the progress made in some countries to contain the epidemic, particularly through: strong political commitment and leadership at the highest levels, including community leadership; effective use of available resources and traditional medicines; successful prevention, care, support and treatment strategies; education and information initiatives; working in partnership with communities, civil society, people living with HIV/AIDS and vulnerable groups; and the active promotion and protection of human rights; and recognizing the importance of sharing and building on our collective and diverse experiences, through regional and international cooperation including North/South, South/South cooperation and triangular cooperation;

28. Acknowledging that resources devoted to combating the epidemic both at the national and international levels are not commensurate with the magnitude of the problem;

29. Recognizing the fundamental importance of strengthening national, regional and subregional capacities to address and effectively combat HIV/AIDS and that this will require increased and sustained human, financial and technical resources through strengthened national action and cooperation and increased regional, subregional and international cooperation;

30. Recognizing that external debt and debt-servicing problems have substantially constrained the capacity of many developing countries, as well as countries with economies in transition, to finance the fight against HIV/AIDS;

31. Affirming the key role played by the family in prevention, care, support and treatment of persons affected and infected by HIV/AIDS, bearing in mind that in different cultural, social and political systems various forms of the family exist;

32. Affirming that beyond the key role played by communities, strong

partnerships among Governments, the United Nations system, intergovernmental organizations, people living with HIV/AIDS and vulnerable groups, medical, scientific and educational institutions, non-governmental organizations, the business sector including generic and research-based pharmaceutical companies, trade unions, media, parliamentarians, foundations, community organizations, faith-based organizations and traditional leaders are important;

33. Acknowledging the particular role and significant contribution of people living with HIV/AIDS, young people and civil society actors in addressing the problem of HIV/AIDS in all its aspects and recognizing that their full involvement and participation in design, planning, implementation and evaluation of programmes is crucial to the development of effective responses to the HIV/AIDS epidemic;

34. Further acknowledging the efforts of international humanitarian organizations combating the epidemic, including among others the volunteers of the International Federation of Red Cross and Red Crescent Societies in the most affected areas all over the world;

35. Commending the leadership role on HIV/AIDS policy and coordination in the United Nations system of the UNAIDS Programme Coordinating Board; noting its endorsement in December 2000 of the Global Strategy Framework for HIV/AIDS, which could assist, as appropriate, Member States and relevant civil society actors in the development of HIV/AIDS strategies, taking into account the particular context of the epidemic in different parts of the world;

36. Solemnly declare our commitment to address the HIV/AIDS crisis by taking action as follows, taking into account the diverse situations and circumstances in different regions and countries throughout the world;

Leadership

Strong leadership at all levels of society is essential for an effective response to the epidemic

Leadership by Governments in combating HIV/AIDS is essential and their efforts should be complemented by the full and active participation of civil society, the business community and the private sector

Leadership involves personal commitment and concrete actions

At the national level

37. By 2003, ensure the development and implementation of multisectoral national strategies and financing plans for combating HIV/AIDS that: address the epidemic in forthright terms; confront

stigma, silence and denial; address gender and age-based dimensions of the epidemic; eliminate discrimination and marginalization; involve partnerships with civil society and the business sector and the full participation of people living with HIV/AIDS, those in vulnerable groups and people mostly at risk, particularly women and young people; are resourced to the extent possible from national budgets without excluding other sources, inter alia international cooperation; fully promote and protect all human rights and fundamental freedoms, including the right to the highest attainable standard of physical and mental health; integrate a gender perspective; and address risk, vulnerability, prevention, care, treatment and support and reduction of the impact of the epidemic; and strengthen health, education and legal system capacity;

38. By 2003, integrate HIV/AIDS prevention, care, treatment and support and impact mitigation priorities into the mainstream of development planning, including in poverty eradication strategies, national budget allocations and sectoral development plans;

At the regional and subregional level

39. Urge and support regional organizations and partners to: be actively involved in addressing the crisis; intensify regional, subregional and interregional cooperation and coordination; and develop regional strategies and responses in support of expanded country level efforts;

40. Support all regional and subregional initiatives on HIV/AIDS including: the International Partnership against AIDS in Africa (IPAA) and the ECA-African Development Forum Consensus and Plan of Action: Leadership to Overcome HIV/ AIDS; the Abuja Declaration and Framework for Action for the Fight Against HIV/AIDS, Tuberculosis and Other Diseases; the CARICOM Pan-Caribbean Partnership Against HIV/AIDS; the ESCAP Regional Call for Action to Fight HIV/ AIDS in Asia and the Pacific; the Baltic Sea Initiative and Action Plan; the Horizontal Technical Cooperation Group on HIV/AIDS in Latin America and the Caribbean; the European Union Programme for Action: Accelerated Action on HIV/AIDS, Malaria and Tuberculosis in the context of poverty reduction;

41. Encourage the development of regional approaches and plans to address HIV/AIDS;

42. Encourage and support local and national organizations to expand and strengthen regional partnerships, coalitions and networks;

43. Encourage the United Nations Economic and Social Council to request the regional commissions within their respective mandates and

resources to support national efforts in their respective regions in combating HIV/AIDS;

At the global level

44. Support greater action and coordination by all relevant United Nations system organizations, including their full participation in the development and implementation of a regularly updated United Nations strategic plan for HIV/AIDS, guided by the principles contained in this Declaration;

45. Support greater cooperation between relevant United Nations system organizations and international organizations combating HIV/AIDS;

46. Foster stronger collaboration and the development of innovative partnerships between the public and private sectors and by 2003, establish and strengthen mechanisms that involve the private sector and civil society partners and people living with HIV/AIDS and vulnerable groups in the fight against HIV/AIDS;

Prevention

Prevention must be the mainstay of our response

47. By 2003, establish time-bound national targets to achieve the internationally agreed global prevention goal to reduce by 2005 HIV prevalence among young men and women aged 15 to 24 in the most affected countries by 25 per cent and by 25 per cent globally by 2010, and to intensify efforts to achieve these targets as well as to challenge gender stereotypes and attitudes, and gender inequalities in relation to HIV/AIDS, encouraging the active involvement of men and boys;

48. By 2003, establish national prevention targets, recognizing and addressing factors leading to the spread of the epidemic and increasing people's vulnerability, to reduce HIV incidence for those identifiable groups, within particular local contexts, which currently have high or increasing rates of HIV infection, or which available public health information indicates are at the highest risk for new infection;

49. By 2005, strengthen the response to HIV/AIDS in the world of work by establishing and implementing prevention and care programmes in public, private and informal work sectors and take measures to provide a supportive workplace environment for people living with HIV/AIDS;

50. By 2005, develop and begin to implement national, regional and international strategies that facilitate access to HIV/AIDS prevention

programmes for migrants and mobile workers, including the provision of information on health and social services;

51. By 2003, implement universal precautions in health-care settings to prevent transmission of HIV infection;

52. By 2005, ensure: that a wide range of prevention programmes which take account of local circumstances, ethics and cultural values, is available in all countries, particularly the most affected countries, including information, education and communication, in languages most understood by communities and respectful of cultures, aimed at reducing risk-taking behaviour and encouraging responsible sexual behaviour, including abstinence and fidelity; expanded access to essential commodities, including male and female condoms and sterile injecting equipment; harm reduction efforts related to drug use; expanded access to voluntary and confidential counselling and testing; safe blood supplies; and early and effective treatment of sexually transmittable infections;

53. By 2005, ensure that at least 90 per cent, and by 2010 at least 95 per cent of young men and women aged 15 to 24 have access to the information, education, including peer education and youth-specific HIV education, and services necessary to develop the life skills required to reduce their vulnerability to HIV infection; in full partnership with youth, parents, families, educators and health-care providers;

54. By 2005, reduce the proportion of infants infected with HIV by 20 per cent, and by 50 per cent by 2010, by: ensuring that 80 per cent of pregnant women accessing antenatal care have information, counselling and other HIV prevention services available to them, increasing the availability of and by providing access for HIV-infected women and babies to effective treatment to reduce mother-to-child transmission of HIV, as well as through effective interventions for HIV-infected women, including voluntary and confidential counselling and testing, access to treatment, especially anti-retroviral therapy and, where appropriate, breast milk substitutes and the provision of a continuum of care;

Care, support and treatment

Care, support and treatment are fundamental elements of an effective response

55. By 2003, ensure that national strategies, supported by regional and international strategies, are developed in close collaboration with the international community, including Governments and relevant intergovernmental organizations as well as with civil society and the business sector, to strengthen health care systems and address factors

affecting the provision of HIV-related drugs, including anti-retroviral drugs, inter alia affordability and pricing, including differential pricing, and technical and health care systems capacity. Also, in an urgent manner make every effort to: provide progressively and in a sustainable manner, the highest attainable standard of treatment for HIV/AIDS, including the prevention and treatment of opportunistic infections, and effective use of quality-controlled anti-retroviral therapy in a careful and monitored manner to improve adherence and effectiveness and reduce the risk of developing resistance; to cooperate constructively in strengthening pharmaceutical policies and practices, including those applicable to generic drugs and intellectual property regimes, in order further to promote innovation and the development of domestic industries consistent with international law;

56. By 2005, develop and make significant progress in implementing comprehensive care strategies to: strengthen family and community-based care including that provided by the informal sector, and health care systems to provide and monitor treatment to people living with HIV/AIDS, including infected children, and to support individuals, households, families and communities affected by HIV/ AIDS; improve the capacity and working conditions of health care personnel, and the effectiveness of supply systems, financing plans and referral mechanisms required to provide access to affordable medicines, including anti-retroviral drugs, diagnostics and related technologies, as well as quality medical, palliative and psycho-social care;

57. By 2003, ensure that national strategies are developed in order to provide psycho-social care for individuals, families, and communities affected by HIV/AIDS;

HIV/AIDS and human rights

Realization of human rights and fundamental freedoms for all is essential to reduce vulnerability to HIV/AIDS

Respect for the rights of people living with HIV/AIDS drives an effective response

58. By 2003, enact, strengthen or enforce as appropriate legislation, regulations and other measures to eliminate all forms of discrimination against, and to ensure the full enjoyment of all human rights and fundamental freedoms by people living with HIV/AIDS and members of vulnerable groups; in particular to ensure their access to, inter alia education, inheritance, employment, health care, social and health services, prevention, support, treatment, information and legal protection, while respecting their privacy and confidentiality; and develop strategies

to combat stigma and social exclusion connected with the epidemic;

59. By 2005, bearing in mind the context and character of the epidemic and that globally women and girls are disproportionately affected by HIV/AIDS, develop and accelerate the implementation of national strategies that: promote the advancement of women and women's full enjoyment of all human rights; promote shared responsibility of men and women to ensure safe sex; empower women to have control over and decide freely and responsibly on matters related to their sexuality to increase their ability to protect themselves from HIV infection;

60. By 2005, implement measures to increase capacities of women and adolescent girls to protect themselves from the risk of HIV infection, principally through the provision of health care and health services, including sexual and reproductive health, and through prevention education that promotes gender equality within a culturally and gender sensitive framework;

61. By 2005, ensure development and accelerated implementation of national strategies for women's empowerment, promotion and protection of women's full enjoyment of all human rights and reduction of their vulnerability to HIV/AIDS through the elimination of all forms of discrimination, as well as all forms of violence against women and girls, including harmful traditional and customary practices, abuse, rape and other forms of sexual violence, battering and trafficking in women and girls;

Reducing vulnerability

The vulnerable must be given priority in the response

Empowering women is essential for reducing vulnerability

62. By 2003, in order to complement prevention programmes that address activities which place individuals at risk of HIV infection, such as risky and unsafe sexual behaviour and injecting drug use, have in place in all countries strategies, policies and programmes that identify and begin to address those factors that make individuals particularly vulnerable to HIV infection, including underdevelopment, economic insecurity, poverty, lack of empowerment of women, lack of education, social exclusion, illiteracy, discrimination, lack of information and/or commodities for self-protection, all types of sexual exploitation of women, girls and boys, including for commercial reasons; such strategies, policies and programmes should address the gender dimension of the epidemic, specify the action that will be taken to address vulnerability and set targets for achievement;

63. By 2003, develop and/or strengthen strategies, policies and programmes, which recognize the importance of the family in reducing vulnerability, inter alia, in educating and guiding children and take account of cultural, religious and ethical factors, to reduce the vulnerability of children and young people by: ensuring access of both girls and boys to primary and secondary education, including on HIV/AIDS in curricula for adolescents; ensuring safe and secure environments, especially for young girls; expanding good quality youth-friendly information and sexual health education and counselling service; strengthening reproductive and sexual health programmes; and involving families and young people in planning, implementing and evaluating HIV/AIDS prevention and care programmes, to the extent possible;

64. By 2003, develop and/or strengthen national strategies, policies and programmes, supported by regional and international initiatives, as appropriate, through a participatory approach, to promote and protect the health of those identifiable groups which currently have high or increasing rates of HIV infection or which public health information indicates are at greatest risk of and most vulnerable to new infection as indicated by such factors as the local history of the epidemic, poverty, sexual practices, drug using behaviour, livelihood, institutional location, disrupted social structures and population movements forced or otherwise;

Children orphaned and made vulnerable by HIV/AIDS

Children orphaned and affected by HIV/AIDS need special assistance

65. By 2003, develop and by 2005 implement national policies and strategies to: build and strengthen governmental, family and community capacities to provide a supportive environment for orphans and girls and boys infected and affected by HIV/AIDS including by providing appropriate counselling and psycho-social support; ensuring their enrolment in school and access to shelter, good nutrition, health and social services on an equal basis with other children; to protect orphans and vulnerable children from all forms of abuse, violence, exploitation, discrimination, trafficking and loss of inheritance;

66. Ensure non-discrimination and full and equal enjoyment of all human rights through the promotion of an active and visible policy of de-stigmatization of children orphaned and made vulnerable by HIV/AIDS;

67. Urge the international community, particularly donor countries, civil society, as well as the private sector to complement effectively

national programmes to support programmes for children orphaned or made vulnerable by HIV/AIDS in affected regions, in countries at high risk and to direct special assistance to sub-Saharan Africa;

Alleviating social and economic impact

To address HIV/AIDS is to invest in sustainable development

68. By 2003, evaluate the economic and social impact of the HIV/AIDS epidemic and develop multisectoral strategies to: address the impact at the individual, family, community and national levels; develop and accelerate the implementation of national poverty eradication strategies to address the impact of HIV/AIDS on household income, livelihoods, and access to basic social services, with special focus on individuals, families and communities severely affected by the epidemic; review the social and economic impact of HIV/AIDS at all levels of society especially on women and the elderly, particularly in their role as caregivers and in families affected by HIV/AIDS and address their special needs; adjust and adapt economic and social development policies, including social protection policies, to address the impact of HIV/AIDS on economic growth, provision of essential economic services, labour productivity, government revenues, and deficit-creating pressures on public resources;

69. By 2003, develop a national legal and policy framework that protects in the workplace the rights and dignity of persons living with and affected by HIV/AIDS and those at the greatest risk of HIV/AIDS in consultation with representatives of employers and workers, taking account of established international guidelines on HIV/AIDS in the workplace;

Research and development

With no cure for HIV/AIDS yet found, further research and development is crucial

70. Increase investment and accelerate research on the development of HIV vaccines, while building national research capacity especially in developing countries, and especially for viral strains prevalent in highly affected regions; in addition, support and encourage increased national and international investment in HIV/AIDS-related research and development including biomedical, operations, social, cultural and behavioural research and in traditional medicine to: improve prevention and therapeutic approaches; accelerate access to prevention, care and treatment and care technologies for HIV/AIDS (and its associated opportunistic infections and malignancies and sexually transmitted diseases), including female controlled methods and

microbicides, and in particular, appropriate, safe and affordable HIV vaccines and their delivery, and to diagnostics, tests, methods to prevent mother-to-child transmission; and improve our understanding of factors which influence the epidemic and actions which address it, inter alia, through increased funding and public/private partnerships; create a conducive environment for research and ensure that it is based on highest ethical standards;

71. Support and encourage the development of national and international research infrastructure, laboratory capacity, improved surveillance systems, data collection, processing and dissemination, and training of basic and clinical researchers, social scientists, health-care providers and technicians, with a focus on the countries most affected by HIV/AIDS, particularly developing countries and those countries experiencing or at risk of rapid expansion of the epidemic;

72. Develop and evaluate suitable approaches for monitoring treatment efficacy, toxicity, side effects, drug interactions, and drug resistance, develop methodologies to monitor the impact of treatment on HIV transmission and risk behaviours;

73. Strengthen international and regional cooperation in particular North/South, South/South and triangular cooperation, related to transfer of relevant technologies, suitable to the environment in prevention and care of HIV/AIDS, the exchange of experiences and best practices, researchers and research findings and strengthen the role of UNAIDS in this process. In this context, encourage that the end results of these cooperative research findings and technologies be owned by all parties to the research, reflecting their relevant contribution and dependent upon their providing legal protection to such findings; and affirm that all such research should be free from bias;

74. By 2003, ensure that all research protocols for the investigation of HIV-related treatment including anti-retroviral therapies and vaccines based on international guidelines and best practices are evaluated by independent committees of ethics, in which persons living with HIV/AIDS and caregivers for anti-retroviral therapy participate;

HIV/AIDS in conflict and disaster affected regions

Conflicts and disasters contribute to the spread of HIV/AIDS

75. By 2003, develop and begin to implement national strategies that incorporate HIV/AIDS awareness, prevention, care and treatment elements into programmes or actions that respond to emergency situations, recognizing that populations destabilized by armed conflict, humanitarian emergencies and natural disasters, including refugees,

internally displaced persons and in particular, women and children, are at increased risk of exposure to HIV infection; and, where appropriate, factor HIV/AIDS components into international assistance programmes;

76. Call on all United Nations agencies, regional and international organizations, as well as non-governmental organizations involved with the provision and delivery of international assistance to countries and regions affected by conflicts, humanitarian crises or natural disasters, to incorporate as a matter of urgency HIV/AIDS prevention, care and awareness elements into their plans and programmes and provide HIV/AIDS awareness and training to their personnel;

77. By 2003, have in place national strategies to address the spread of HIV among national uniformed services, where this is required, including armed forces and civil defence force and consider ways of using personnel from these services who are educated and trained in HIV/AIDS awareness and prevention to assist with HIV/ AIDS awareness and prevention activities including participation in emergency, humanitarian, disaster relief and rehabilitation assistance;

78. By 2003, ensure the inclusion of HIV/AIDS awareness and training, including a gender component, into guidelines designed for use by defence personnel and other personnel involved in international peacekeeping operations while also continuing with ongoing education and prevention efforts, including pre-deployment orientation, for these personnel;

Resources

The HIV/AIDS challenge cannot be met without new, additional and sustained resources

79. Ensure that the resources provided for the global response to address HIV/AIDS are substantial, sustained and geared towards achieving results;

80. By 2005, through a series of incremental steps, reach an overall target of annual expenditure on the epidemic of between US$ 7 billion and US$ 10 billion in low and middle-income countries and those countries experiencing or at risk of experiencing rapid expansion for prevention, care, treatment, support and mitigation of the impact of HIV/AIDS, and take measures to ensure that needed resources are made available, particularly from donor countries and also from national budgets, bearing in mind that resources of the most affected countries are seriously limited;

81. Call on the international community, where possible, to provide assistance for HIV/AIDS prevention, care and treatment in developing countries on a grant basis;

82. Increase and prioritize national budgetary allocations for HIV/AIDS programmes as required and ensure that adequate allocations are made by all ministries and other relevant stakeholders;

83. Urge the developed countries that have not done so to strive to meet the targets of 0.7 per cent of their gross national product for overall official development assistance and the targets of earmarking of 0.15 per cent to 0.20 per cent of gross national product as official development assistance for least developed countries as agreed, as soon as possible, taking into account the urgency and gravity of the HIV/AIDS epidemic;

84. Urge the international community to complement and supplement efforts of developing countries that commit increased national funds to fight the HIV/AIDS epidemic through increased international development assistance, particularly those countries most affected by HIV/AIDS, particularly in Africa, especially in sub-Saharan Africa, the Caribbean, countries at high risk of expansion of the HIV/AIDS epidemic and other affected regions whose resources to deal with the epidemic are seriously limited;

85. Integrate HIV/AIDS actions in development assistance programmes and poverty eradication strategies as appropriate and encourage the most effective and transparent use of all resources allocated;

86. Call on the international community and invite civil society and the private sector to take appropriate measures to help alleviate the social and economic impact of HIV/AIDS in the most affected developing countries;

87. Without further delay implement the enhanced Heavily Indebted Poor Country (HIPC) Initiative and agree to cancel all bilateral official debts of HIPC countries as soon as possible, especially those most affected by HIV/AIDS, in return for their making demonstrable commitments to poverty eradication and urge the use of debt service savings to finance poverty eradication programmes, particularly for HIV/AIDS prevention, treatment, care and support and other infections;

88. Call for speedy and concerted action to address effectively the debt problems of least developed countries, low-income developing countries, and middle-income developing countries, particularly those affected by HIV/AIDS, in a comprehensive, equitable, development-

oriented and durable way through various national and international measures designed to make their debt sustainable in the long term and thereby to improve their capacity to deal with the HIV/AIDS epidemic, including, as appropriate, existing orderly mechanisms for debt reduction, such as debt swaps for projects aimed at the prevention, care and treatment of HIV/AIDS;

89. Encourage increased investment in HIV/AIDS-related research, nationally, regionally and internationally, in particular for the development of sustainable and affordable prevention technologies, such as vaccines and microbicides, and encourage the proactive preparation of financial and logistic plans to facilitate rapid access to vaccines when they become available;

90. Support the establishment, on an urgent basis, of a global HIV/AIDS and health fund to finance an urgent and expanded response to the epidemic based on an integrated approach to prevention, care, support and treatment and to assist Governments inter alia in their efforts to combat HIV/AIDS with due priority to the most affected countries, notably in sub-Saharan Africa and the Caribbean and to those countries at high risk, mobilize contributions to the fund from public and private sources with a special appeal to donor countries, foundations, the business community including pharmaceutical companies, the private sector, philanthropists and wealthy individuals;

91. By 2002, launch a worldwide fund-raising campaign aimed at the general public as well as the private sector, conducted by UNAIDS with the support and collaboration of interested partners at all levels, to contribute to the global HIV/ AIDS and health fund;

92. Direct increased funding to national, regional and subregional commissions and organizations to enable them to assist Governments at the national, subregional and regional level in their efforts to respond to the crisis;

93. Provide the UNAIDS co-sponsoring agencies and the UNAIDS secretariat with the resources needed to work with countries in support of the goals of this Declaration;

Follow-up

Maintaining the momentum and monitoring progress are essential

At the national level

94. Conduct national periodic reviews involving the participation of civil society, particularly people living with HIV/AIDS, vulnerable

groups and caregivers, of progress achieved in realizing these commitments and identify problems and obstacles to achieving progress and ensure wide dissemination of the results of these reviews;

95. Develop appropriate monitoring and evaluation mechanisms to assist with follow-up in measuring and assessing progress, develop appropriate monitoring and evaluation instruments, with adequate epidemiological data;

96. By 2003, establish or strengthen effective monitoring systems, where appropriate, for the promotion and protection of human rights of people living with HIV/AIDS;

At the regional level

97. Include HIV/AIDS and related public health concerns as appropriate on the agenda of regional meetings at the ministerial and Head of State and Government level;

98. Support data collection and processing to facilitate periodic reviews by regional commissions and/or regional organizations of progress in implementing regional strategies and addressing regional priorities and ensure wide dissemination of the results of these reviews;

99. Encourage the exchange between countries of information and experiences in implementing the measures and commitments contained in this Declaration, and in particular facilitate intensified South-South and triangular cooperation;

At the global level

100. Devote sufficient time and at least one full day of the annual General Assembly session to review and debate a report of the Secretary-General on progress achieved in realizing the commitments set out in this Declaration, with a view to identifying problems and constraints and making recommendations on action needed to make further progress;

101. Ensure that HIV/AIDS issues are included on the agenda of all appropriate United Nations conferences and meetings;

102. Support initiatives to convene conferences, seminars, workshops, training programmes and courses to follow up issues raised in this Declaration and in this regard encourage participation in and wide dissemination of the outcomes of: the forthcoming Dakar Conference on Access to Care for HIV Infection; the Sixth International Congress on AIDS in Asia and the Pacific; the XII International Conference on AIDS and Sexually Transmitted Infections in Africa; the XIV

International Conference on AIDS, Barcelona; the Xth International Conference on People Living with HIV/AIDS, Port of Spain; the II Forum and III Conference of the Latin American and the Caribbean Horizontal Technical Cooperation on HIV/AIDS and Sexually Transmitted Infections, La Habana; the Vth International Conference on Home and Community Care for Persons Living with HIV/AIDS, Changmai, Thailand;

103. Explore, with a view to improving equity in access to essential drugs, the feasibility of developing and implementing, in collaboration with non-governmental organizations and other concerned partners, systems for voluntary monitoring and reporting of global drug prices;

We recognize and express our appreciation to those who have led the effort to raise awareness of the HIV/AIDS epidemic and to deal with its complex challenges;

We look forward to strong leadership by Governments, and concerted efforts with full and active participation of the United Nations, the entire multilateral system, civil society, the business community and private sector;

And finally, we call on all countries to take the necessary steps to implement this Declaration, in strengthened partnership and cooperation with other multilateral and bilateral partners and with civil society.

FROM THE UNIVERSAL DECLARATION OF HUMAN RIGHTS

Adopted and proclaimed by General Assembly resolution 217 A (III) of 10 December 1948.

Article 3.

Everyone has the right to life, liberty and security of person.

Article 19.

Everyone has the right to freedom of opinion and expression; this right includes freedom to hold opinions without interference and to seek, receive and impart information and ideas through any media and regardless of frontiers.

Article 25.

(1) Everyone has the right to a standard of living adequate for the health and well-being of himself and of his family, including food, clothing, housing and medical care and necessary social services, and the right to security in the event of unemployment, sickness, disability, widowhood, old age or other lack of livelihood in circumstances beyond his control.

(2) Motherhood and childhood are entitled to special care and assistance. All children, whether born in or out of wedlock, shall enjoy the same social protection.

FROM THE INTERNATIONAL COVENANT ON ECONOMIC, SOCIAL AND CULTURAL RIGHTS

Adopted and opened for signature, ratification and accession by General Assembly resolution 2200 A (XXI) of 16 December 1966

Article 12

1.   The States Parties to the present Covenant recognize the right of everyone to the enjoyment of the highest attainable standard of physical and mental health.

2.   The steps to be taken by the States Parties to the present Covenant to achieve the full realization of this right shall include those necessary for:

(a) The provision for the reduction of the stillbirth-rate and infant mortality and for the healthy development of the child;

(b) The improvement of all aspects of environmental and industrial hygiene;

(c) The prevention, treatment and control of epidemic, endemic, occupational and other diseases;

(d) The creation of conditions which would assure all medical service and medical attention in the event of sickness.

FROM THE GENERAL COMMENT NO. 14

COMMITTEE ON ECONOMIC, SOCIAL AND CULTURAL RIGHTS
Twenty-second session, Geneva, 25 April-12 May 2000

The right to the highest attainable standard of health
(article 12 of the International Covenant on Economic, Social
and Cultural Rights)

1. Health is a fundamental human right indispensable for the exercise of other human rights. Every human being is entitled to the enjoyment of the highest attainable standard of health conducive to living a life in dignity. The realization of the right to health may be pursued through numerous, complementary approaches, such as the formulation of health policies, or the implementation of health programmes developed by the World Health Organization (WHO), or the adoption of specific legal instruments which are legally enforceable (1).

3. The right to health is closely related to and dependent upon the realization of other human rights, as contained in the International Bill of Rights, including the rights to food, housing, work, education, human dignity, life, non-discrimination, equality, the prohibition against torture, privacy, access to information, and the freedoms of association, assembly and movement. These and other rights and freedoms address integral components of the right to health.

9. The notion of "the highest attainable standard of health" in article 12.1 takes into account both the individual's biological and socio-economic preconditions and a State's available resources. There are a number of aspects which cannot be addressed solely within the relationship between States and individuals; in particular, good health cannot be ensured by a State, nor can States provide protection against every possible cause of human ill health. Thus, genetic factors, individual susceptibility to ill health and the adoption of unhealthy or risky lifestyles may play an important role with respect to an individual's health.

Consequently, the right to health must be understood as a right to the enjoyment of a variety of facilities, goods, services and conditions necessary for the realization of the highest attainable standard of health.

10. Since the adoption of the two International Covenants in 1966 the world health situation has changed dramatically and the notion of health has undergone substantial changes and has also widened in scope. More determinants of health are being taken into consideration, such as resource distribution and gender differences. A wider definition of health also takes into account such socially-related concerns as violence and armed conflict. (2 www.unhchr.ch/tbs/doc.nsf/8e9c603f 486cdf83802566f8003870e7/40d009901358b0e2 c1256915005090be? OpenDocument) Moreover, formerly unknown diseases, such as Human Immunodeficiency Virus and Acquired Immunodeficiency Syndrome (HIV/AIDS), and others that have become more widespread, such as cancer, as well as the rapid growth of the world population, have created new obstacles for the realization of the right to health which need to be taken into account when interpreting article 12.

11. The Committee interprets the right to health, as defined in article 12.1, as an inclusive right extending not only to timely and appropriate health care but also to the underlying determinants of health, such as access to safe and potable water and adequate sanitation, an adequate supply of safe food, nutrition and housing, healthy occupational and environmental conditions, and access to health-related education and information, including on sexual and reproductive health. A further important aspect is the participation of the population in all health-related decision-making at the community, national and international levels.

Article 12.2 (c). The right to prevention, treatment and control of diseases

16. "The prevention, treatment and control of epidemic, endemic, occupational and other diseases" (art. 12.2 (c)) requires the establishment of prevention and education programmes for behaviour-related health concerns such as sexually transmitted diseases, in particular HIV/AIDS, and those adversely affecting sexual and reproductive health, and the promotion of social determinants of good health, such as environmental safety, education, economic development and gender equity.

The right to treatment includes the creation of a system of urgent medical care in cases of accidents, epidemics and similar health hazards, and the provision of disaster relief and humanitarian assistance in emergency situations. The control of diseases refers to States' individual and joint efforts to, inter alia, make available relevant technologies, using and improving epidemiological surveillance and data collection on a disaggregated basis, the implementation or enhancement of immunization programmes and other strategies of infectious disease control.

18. By virtue of article 2.2 and article 3, the Covenant proscribes any discrimination in access to health care and underlying determinants of health, as well as to means and entitlements for their procurement, on the grounds of race, colour, sex, language, religion, political or other opinion, national or social origin, property, birth, physical or mental disability, health status (including HIV/AIDS), sexual orientation and civil, political, social or other status, which has the intention or effect of nullifying or impairing the equal enjoyment or exercise of the right to health. The Committee stresses that many measures, such as most strategies and programmes designed to eliminate health-related discrimination, can be pursued with minimum resource implications through the adoption, modification or abrogation of legislation or the dissemination of information. The Committee recalls General Comment No. 3, paragraph 12, which states that even in times of severe resource constraints, the vulnerable members of society must be protected by the adoption of relatively low-cost targeted programmes.

23. States parties should provide a safe and supportive environment for adolescents, that ensures the opportunity to participate in decisions affecting their health, to build life-skills, to acquire appropriate information, to receive counselling and to negotiate the health-behaviour choices they make. The realization of the right to health of adolescents is dependent on the development of youth-friendly health care, which respects confidentiality and privacy and includes appropriate sexual and reproductive health services.

24. In all policies and programmes aimed at guaranteeing the right to health of children and adolescents their best interests shall be a primary consideration.

NOTES

1. For example, the principle of non-discrimination in relation to health facilities, goods and services is legally enforceable in numerous national jurisdictions.
2. Common article 3 of the Geneva Conventions for the protection of war victims (1949); Additional Protocol I (1977) relating to the Protection of Victims of International Armed Conflicts, art. 75 (2) (a); Additional Protocol II (1977) relating to the Protection of Victims of Non-International Armed Conflicts, art. 4(a).

FROM THE INTERNATIONAL COVENANT ON CIVIL AND POLITICAL RIGHTS

Adopted and opened for signature, ratification and accession by General Assembly resolution 2200 A (XXI) of 16 December1966

Article 9

1. Everyone has the right to liberty and security of person. No one shall be subjected to arbitrary arrest or detention. No one shall be deprived of his liberty except on such grounds and in accordance with such procedure as are established by law.

2. Anyone who is arrested shall be informed, at the time of arrest, of the reasons for his arrest and shall be promptly informed of any charges against him.

3. Anyone arrested or detained on a criminal charge shall be brought promptly before a judge or other officer authorized by law to exercise judicial power and shall be entitled to trial within a reasonable time or to release. It shall not be the general rule that persons awaiting trial shall be detained in custody, but release may be subject to guarantees to appear for trial, at any other stage of the judicial proceedings, and, should occasion arise, for execution of the judgement.

4. Anyone who is deprived of his liberty by arrest or detention shall be entitled to take proceedings before a court, in order that court may decide without delay on the lawfulness of his detention and order his release if the detention is not lawful.

5. Anyone who has been the victim of unlawful arrest or detention shall have an enforceable right to compensation.

Article 17

1. No one shall be subjected to arbitrary or unlawful interference with

his privacy, family, home or correspondence, nor to unlawful attacks on his honour and reputation.

2. Everyone has the right to the protection of the law against such interference or attacks.

Article 26

All persons are equal before the law and are entitled without any discrimination to the equal protection of the law. In this respect, the law shall prohibit any discrimination and guarantee to all persons equal and effective protection against discrimination on any ground such as race, colour, sex, language, religion, political or other opinion, national or social origin, property, birth or other status.

FROM THE EUROPEAN CONVENTION FOR THE PROTECTION OF HUMAN RIGHTS AND FUNDAMENTAL FREEDOMS

Rome, 4 November 1950
as amended by Protocol No. 11 (ETS No. 155).

Article 5

1. Everyone has the right to liberty and security of person.

No one shall be deprived of his liberty save in the following cases and in accordance with a procedure prescribed by law:

(a) the lawful detention of a person after conviction by a competent court;

(b) the lawful arrest or detention of a person for non-compliance with the lawful order of a court or in order to secure the fulfilment of any obligation prescribed by law;

(c) the lawful arrest or detention of a person effected for the purpose of bringing him before the competent legal authority of reasonable suspicion of having committed and offence or when it is reasonably considered necessary to prevent his committing an offence or fleeing after having done so;

(d) the detention of a minor by lawful order for the purpose of educational supervision or his lawful detention for the purpose of bringing him before the competent legal authority;

(e) the lawful detention of persons for the prevention of the spreading of infectious diseases, of persons of unsound mind, alcoholics or drug addicts, or vagrants;

(f) the lawful arrest or detention of a person to prevent his effecting an unauthorized entry into the country or of a person against whom action is being taken with a view to deportation or extradition.

Article 8

1. Everyone has the right to respect for his private and family life, his home and his correspondence.

FROM THE INTERNATIONAL CONVENTION AGAINST ILLICIT TRAFFIC IN NARCOTIC DRUGS AND PSYCHOTROPIC SUBSTANCES

adopted by the Conference at its 6th plenary meeting, on 19 December 1988.

Article 14

MEASURES TO ERADICATE ILLICIT CULTIVATION OF NARCOTIC PLANTS AND TO ELIMINATE ILLICIT DEMAND FOR NARCOTIC DRUGS AND PSYCHOTROPIC SUBSTANCES

1. Any measures taken pursuant to this Convention by Parties shall not be less stringent than the provisions applicable to the eradication of illicit cultivation of plants containing narcotic and psychotropic substances and to the elimination of illicit demand for narcotic drugs and psychotropic substances under the provisions of the 1961 Convention, the 1961 Convention as amended and the 1971 Convention.

2. Each Party shall take appropriate measures to prevent illicit cultivation of and to eradicate plants containing narcotic or psychotropic substances, such as opium poppy, coca bush and cannabis plants, cultivated illicitly in its territory. The measures adopted shall respect fundamental human rights and shall take due account of traditional licit uses, where there is historic evidence of such use, as well as the protection of the environment.

3. (a) The Parties may co-operate to increase the effectiveness of eradication efforts. Such co-operation may, *inter alia*, include support, when appropriate, for integrated rural development leading

to economically viable alternatives to illicit cultivation. Factors such as access to markets, the availability of resources and prevailing socio-economic conditions should be taken into account before such rural development programmes are implemented. The Parties may agree on any other appropriate measures of co-operation.

(b) The Parties shall also facilitate the exchange of scientific and technical information and the conduct of research concerning eradication.

(c) Whenever they have common frontiers, the Parties shall seek to co-operate in eradication programmes in their respective areas along those frontiers.

4. The Parties shall adopt appropriate measures aimed at eliminating or reducing illicit demand for narcotic drugs and psychotropic substances, with a view to reducing human suffering and eliminating financial incentives for illicit traffic. These measures may be based, *inter alia*, on the recommendations of the United Nations, specialized agencies of the United Nations such as the World Health Organization, and other competent international organizations, and on the Comprehensive Multidisciplinary Outline adopted by the International Conference on Drug Abuse and Illicit Trafficking, held in 1987, as it pertains to governmental and non-governmental agencies and private efforts in the fields of prevention, treatment and rehabilitation. The Parties may enter into bilateral or multilateral agreements or arrangements aimed at eliminating or reducing illicit demand for narcotic drugs and psychotropic substances.

FROM THE INTERNATIONAL GUIDELINES ON HIV/AIDS AND HUMAN RIGHTS

adopted at the Second International Consultation on HIV/AIDS and Human Rights, Geneva, 23–25 September 1996.

Guideline 3

States should review and reform public health laws to ensure that they adequately address public health issues raised by HIV/AIDS, that their provisions applicable to casually transmitted diseases are not inappropriately applied to HIV/AIDS and that they are consistent with international human rights obligations.

Guidleline 4

States should review and reform criminal laws and correctional systems to ensure that they are consistent with international human rights obligations and are not misused in the context of HIV/AIDS or targeted against vulnerable groups.

Part 5
Glossary

Addiction[1] – a dependence on a substance such as alcohol or other drugs or a dependence on an activity, to the point that stopping it is very difficult and causes severe physical and mental reactions. Addiction to a drug is a pattern of compulsive drug use characterized by a continued craving, as for example for an opioid and the need to use the opioid for effects other than pain relief.

AIDS – a disease due to infection with the human immunodeficiency virus (HIV). AIDS is an acronym for Acquired Immuno Deficiency Syndrome.

Criminal law – a general term that is used in regard to the law of crimes and their punishment. These laws are written and passed by the appropriate governmental institutions (Congress, Parliament) and make certain behavior illegal and punishable by fines and/or imprisonment.

Crime – an act or the commision of an act that is forbidden by law. Detailed legal definitions of "crime" vary from country to country and are usually found in Criminal Codes or other criminal statutes.

Decriminalization policy – this term can be used to describe another type of drug policy, where personal use, posession, cultivation of drugs, are defined as illegal, but entail only nominal fines.

Drug policy – a general term, describing rules, legislation and practice of governmental agencies towards drugs.

Drug-related harm – negative consequences of drug use, including, but not limited to: transmission of blood-borne and other infections, vein diseases, overdoses, loss of work, etc.

Hepatitis – inflammation of the liver.

Hepatitis C – inflammation of the liver due to the HCV (hepatitis C virus), which is spread by blood. The damage the virus causes to the liver can lead to cirrhosis and cancer. There is no vaccine against this type of hepatitis. It is diagnosed by a blood test.

HIV – Human Immunodeficiency Virus, the retrovirus that causes AIDS. It is now generally accepted that the virus was first discovered in 1983 – 1984 by French physician Luc Monatagnier and his team at the Pasteur Institute.

Human rights – inalienable basic rights intended to protect all people from cruel and inhumane treatment, threats to their lives, and persecution. Usually referred to rights found in the Universal Declaration of Human Rights (UN General Assembly Declaration of December 10, 1948) where definitions for the civil, political, economic, social, and cultural rights of human beings are provided.

Legalization – a vague term, its meaning can range from legal provision of drugs to a person, known to use drugs to the open public access to all drugs.

Overdose – a term used to describe excessive consumption of drugs that leads to negative health consequences, including death.

Possession of drugs without intent to sell – countries with prohibitionists' drug laws this term may be used to distinguish between criminal behavior – sale of substances that are considered to be illicit, and possession with the intent to sell, and possession for one's own use.

Pragmatic approach to disease prevention – an approach to public health which is mainly based on pragmatism and disease prevention, as opposed to the one based on political interests of governmental agencies involved.

Privacy – broad philosophical conception, that is interconnected with the conception of human dignity.

Prohibition policy – a type of drug policy, under which the cultivation, production, use, posession and sale of drugs are all regarded as a criminal offence. Can also be referred to as a restrictive policy that maintans legal restrictions against the non-medical use or sale addicting drugs.

Right to privacy – one of the fundamental human rights, protected by the Universal Declaration of Human Rights, the International Covenant on Civil and Political Rights and other international treaties. The right to privacy includes freedom from unwarranted searches and seizures, collecting and handling personal information (including health information), privacy of one's territory (whether it is house, working environment, public place), etc.

Supply reduction policies – types of drug policy, where the main focus is made on reducing the availability of illicit drugs.

WHO (World Health Organization) – a specialized agency of the United Nations, dedicated to the promotion of health, defined as "a state of complete physical, mental and social well-being and not merely the absence of disease or infirmity". Homepage: www.who.int.

UNAIDS – Joint United Nations Programme on HIV/AIDS (UNAIDS). Since April1999, the programme includes seven co-sponsoring agencies: UNICEF, UNDP, UNFPA, UNESCO, WHO, the World Bank and UNDCP. The goal of UNAIDS is to catalyse, strengthen and orchestrate the unique expertise, resources, and networks of influence that each of these organizations offers in order to reduce the spread of HIV/AIDS in the world, as well as its impact. Homepage: www.unaids.org.

NOTES

[1] As defined in the Online Dictionary for Medical Terms, www.medterms.com (date assessed October 02, 2001).